Nature's Weeds Native Medicine

Native American Herbal Secrets

Marie Miczak, D.Sc., Ph.D.

LOTUS
PRESS

Published by: Lotus Press
P.O. Box 325, Twin Lakes, WI 53181 USA

DISCLAIMER

The information contained in this book is provided to be used in conjunction with the guidance of your professional health care provider. The remedies described here are neither advice or prescriptions, but the historical and current uses of herbs by Native American peoples. Based largely on empirical evidence, these ideas involve just one facet of the total health care picture. Any remedy from any source should be employed with caution, common sense and the approval of your professional health care provider.

Design – Cover and Page layout: Linda Khristal
Illustrations: Richard Koehler
Dr. Miczak's Photograph: Joseph Yawboh Miczak
Cover Photograph: Images® copyright 1999 PhotoDisc, Inc.

First Edition, 1999

Printed in the United States of America
Library of Congress Cataloging-inPublication Data
Miczak, Marie

ISBN: Library of Congress
978-0-9149-5548-1   Catalogue No. 98-75821

Published by: Lotus Press
P.O. Box 325, Twin Lakes, Wisconsin 53181 USA
e-mail: lotuspress@lotuspress.com
website: www.lotuspress.com

For Mom and Dad...

For all you've given me.

***Great Mystery*...**

All you bestow upon us

Astound and surprise...

And yet you are taken for granted

Simultaneously...

We watch in bewilderment and amazement

Catching a glimpse of what was

And what is yet to be

Now we must thank you for all you have given

Unconditionally...

You give and you give

Thank you for letting us dip into your garden

We are blessed...

With your healing powers.

Roberta Braun Shapiro

TABLE OF CONTENTS

Preface x

Foreword xii

CHAPTER ONE

THE HISTORY OF THE USE OF HERBS BY EARLY NATIVE AMERICANS

Old World Medicine 1

Use of Herbs in North America 2

Native Healing Traditions Practiced Today 7

CHAPTER TWO

THE MEDICINE POUCH...

...Your Guide to Indigenous Herbs 11
Beechnut 14 – Beebalm 15 – Black Birch 16 – Blue Cohosh 17 – Cattail 19 – Wild Cherry 20 – Corn 21 – Dock 22 – Echinacea 23 – Elderberry 25 – Goldenseal 26 – False & Solomon's Seal 27 – Hydrangea 28 – Juniper 29 – Jerusalem Artichoke 30 – Maple32 – Mint 33 – Nettle 35 – Plantain 36 – Red Clover 37 – Red Raspberry 38 – Sage 39– Willow Bark 41

Growing Your Own Native Herbs 43 – Harvesting & Drying 45 – Framing Out Your Garden 46 – Herbal Planting Chart 49 – Planting Your Garden 51 – Maintaining Your Garden 52

CHAPTER THREE

MAKING YOUR OWN HERBAL FORMULAS

Overview of Herbal Remedy Preparation 53

Basic Herbal Products 56 – Infusions 56 – Decoctions 56 – Syrups 57 – Tinctures & Vinegars 57 – Infused Oils & Ointments 58 – Poultices & Compresses 59

Herbal Recipes for: Skin, Hair & Body Care 61

Skin Care 61 – Corn Meal Bath Scrub 61 – Herbal Facial Cleanser 62 – Antiseptic Pine Acne Cleanser 62 – Skin Healing Wash 63 – Witchhazel Toner 63 – Gentle Mint Toner 64 – Most Gentle Rose Toner 64 – Natural Native Moisturizer 65 – Native Skin Nourisher 65 – Clover Blossom Bath Oil 65 – Calendula After Bath Oil 66 – Natural Deodorant 66 – Natural Athlete's Foot Spray 66 – Natural Douche 67 – Natural Tooth Powder 68 – Natural Mouthwash 68

Natural Native Hair Care 69 – Soapweed Natural Shampoo 69– Shine Enhancing Shampoo 69– Maple Deep Conditioning Treatment 70 – Pumpkin Conditioner 70 – Hair Darkening Tonic 71 – Fresh Mint Hair Rinse 71 – Hair Restoring Rinse 71 – Hair Strengthening Conditioner 72 – Hot Oil Treatment for Dry, Breaking Hair 73 – Mineral Hair Masque 73 – Light Hair Pomade 74

Special Time-Honored Remedies 75

Little Crow's Soothing Salve 75 – Plantain Leaf Salve 76 – Comfrey Salve 76 – Red Clover Salve 77

Recipes for the Home   **78**

Pine Room Freshener 78 – Aromatic Pine Blend 79
– Cedarwood Pouch Blend 80 – Pine Needle Fire Place
Sticks 80 – Cattail Aromatic Pillow 81 – Sweet Grass Blocks
81 – Pine Needle Blocks 82 – Cedarwood Blocks 82 –
Naturally Died & Scented Baskets 83 – Scented Stones 84

CHAPTER FOUR

FOOD IS MEDICINE...

...and Medicine is Food   **85**

Corn Pancakes with Maple Syrup 86 – Fried Cinnamon
Apples 87 – Oh-No-Kwa (Hominy Grits) 88 – Sapan
(Lenape – White Cornmeal Gruel) 88 – Anakee's Mulberry
Muffins 89 – Corn Bread (squares or muffins) 89 – Pumpkin
Bread 90 – Grandmother "Hoosh's" Light Rolls 91 –
Cherokee Fry Bread 92 – Broiled Tomatoes 92 – Baked
Sweet Potatoes 93 – Baked Pumpkin 93 – Aunt Lizzy's
Potatoes 94 – Mom's Crookneck Squash 95 – Pow Wow
Corn Soup 95 – Birch Bark Chicken 96 – Roast Corn 96 –
Skewered Scallops 97 – Roast Cornish Game Hen w/
Cornbread-Oyster Stuffing 97 – Pumpkin or Winter Squash
Pie 98 – Snow Ice Cream 99 – Maple Walnut Cookies 99

Refreshing Herbal Teas   **100**

Native Women's Blend 101 – Natural Fertility Blend 101 –
Native Pregnancy Tea 102 – Breastmilk Builder 102
– Teepee Creepers Pleaser 102 – Midday Energizer 103 –
Cold Chaser Blend 103 – Iron Tonic 104 – Tummy Soother

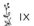

104 − Natural Calm Tea Blend 105 − Sunrise Herb Tea Blend
105 − Slimming Tea Blend 106 − Natural Brain Power Blend
106 − Blues Chaser Blend 106

Native American Kitchen Remedies   108

Onions for Colds and Fever 108 − Octagon Soap for Skin
Irritations and Poison Ivy 109 − Aesthetic Badge to Ward Off
Disease 109

Glossary   110

Native Herbs − Quick Reference   113

Conversion Chart   118

References and Resources   119

Helpful Books 119 − Herbal Supplies 119 − Native American
News Journals and Magazines 121 − Native American Clothing
and Crafts 122

Index   123

ILLUSTRATIONS

Page 11   *Corn Husk Mask* − Used in the healing ceremonies of the
             Iroquois.
Page 42   *False Face Mask* − Used by secret medicine societies of the
             Iroquois.
Page 44   *Corn Picking Pack Basket* − Split Ash, Mohawk
Page 60   *Southwestern Pottery Jars* − Lizard design
Page 83   *Porcupine Quill & Split Ash Baskets* − Iroquois

Preface

In any endeavor, it is often those unseen individuals who most contribute to the success of any viable work. My first and best teachers were my parents. Neither had ever gone to college, but they instilled in me an insatiable desire to investigate all forms of scientific reasoning. By taking me to museums, parks, zoos and cultural exhibits at a very young age, I was inspired to keep asking questions, keep seeking answers. Their confidence in my abilities never wavered as I was often encouraged by my father to "Shoot for the Moon, because who knows, you might just end up among the stars." My mother, to this day, remains one of my most loyal supporters and has taught me perhaps the most about human nature. My husband of more than 19 years has also exposed me to a world of discovery. With our children, we have visited scientific exhibits all over the country to hopefully instill in them that same desire to learn. My children have been very supportive, allowing me to focus on projects and even offering much needed assistance towards completion.

When I first sought resources to develop courses in botanical medicine for Brookdale Community College, I turned to my alma mater, Rutgers University College of Pharmacy. The college's dean, Dr. Bartly Sciarrone, took the time to answer my questions and refer me to the professor who taught pharmacognosy, the study of medicines derived from plants and natural resources. Dr. Philip Babcock introduced me to the likes of James Duke and Varro Tyler whose texts were standard reference for the subject. Dr. Babcock told me that pharmacognosy is no longer being taught at many pharmacy colleges, because so much of the medication today is synthetic or chemically manufactured. All the same, up to 40% of all medication contains some herbal or natural component even now. Dean Babcock lamented that it is ironic that at a time when more of the public is using herbal preparations of all sorts, less and less time is being spent in the classroom on pharmacognosy. I'd like to thank both deans Sciarrone and Babcock for their encouragement, support and help throughout my professional career.

Two people who have also impacted my projects, specifically in computer literacy and utilization, are Roberta and Ken Shapiro. This couple has unselfishly given of their time to help me become more productive in my research, writing and communications. Ken David Shapiro, with his vast knowledge of computers from the ground up, has kept my programs running smoothly and introduced me to new applications which have helped me to expand my horizons. For his guidance and assistance, I am truly grateful.

Most of all I have to acknowledge the Creator, Jehovah God, in all of his wisdom in providing mankind with such a wide array of plants of every description for sustenance, health and healing. Even more gracious is God's granting of our inherent curiosity and mental capacity to explore and learn more about the riches of the earth at our very doorstep, the healing herbs.

FOREWORD

Today, perhaps more than ever, people are looking for alternatives to orthodox medicine's toxic drugs and invasive surgeries. In fact, according to the World Health Organization (WHO), nearly two thirds of the world's population relies regularly on herbs and botanicals. In England and France especially, doctors routinely write prescriptions using herbal medicines for everything from self-limiting illnesses to severe infections with great success. Also worthy of note is the fact that in 1993 the New England Journal of Medicine reported a study which showed approximately 34% of Americans using at least one form of alternative health care during 1990 including plant based medicine. Since then these numbers have grown steadily as evidenced by Harvard Medical School, Tufts, and Duke Universities researching natural medicines in an attempt to address the public's increased demand for knowledge about herbal modalities.

Major pharmaceutical companies such as Merck & Co. have been following suit by purchasing 1 square mile of Central American Rain Forest for the purpose of studying the vast variety of plants and animals existing there, many of which are unclassified or cataloged. Pharmacognosy, or the study of medicines derived from plants and natural sources, despite reports to the contrary, is making a resurgence. While not sounding like a very large terrain to investigate, keep in mind that one square mile of Central American Rainforest contains more biodiversity than the entire state of New York. Adding to the urgency of this mission are the local medicine men and women who are quickly passing away without passing on this centuries acquired knowledge of the use of these herbs to younger progeny. Keep in mind that many herbs are used by native tribes in complex combinations, synergizing their effects beyond what may be detected in the pharmacologist's laboratory. Differences in altitude, growing conditions and soil compositions will concurrently effect the plants medicinal properties causing wide variations within the same species. All of these issues are known, however, by the native healers who have harvested and prepared these herbs for health and healing for centuries.

Highly obscure are the ancient herbal medicinal formulas used by the first inhabitants of North America. Native American Herbal Secrets will present many traditional healing herbs of the indigenous peoples of the United States. Rather than disappearing, these native medicinal practices have been absorbed into the melting pot known broadly as American folk medicine. Tied into the cultural myths and traditions, this book will clearly illuminate the wisdom of our forefathers as healers, medicine men and women as well as midwives. Unlike other titles which have attempted to cover this subject, this publication offers specific insights, actual detailed formulas and an intimate view of the Native American's perception concerning the curative use of herbs.

It is the aim of this book to provide the reader with in-depth subject material easily applied for modern use. Acknowledging that herbs are not a panacea, there is great care taken in this book to advise when interactions may occur and what botanicals should not be used by individuals with specific preexisting medical conditions. As a member of A Ph A's Academy of Pharmaceutical Science and Research, Dr. Miczak will be able to show how these herbs are being validated by modern scientific research today as well as their safe and judicious applications. As a Native American, she brings with her personal experiences and an insider's view of her tribe's healing techniques for better health. This rare but valuable information on the botanical formulas implemented by the first Americans qualifies as the historical heritage of every American.

CHAPTER ONE

HISTORY OF THE USE OF HERBS BY EARLY NATIVE AMERICANS

Old World Medicine

Since the twilight of unrecorded history, man's quest to gain control over the invisible forces dominating his life and well being has caused him to explore, experiment and note the natural medicinal values of plants and animals found on his native soil. The earliest written documentation of medicines dates back to about 3,500 years ago. The successive civilizations of the Tigris-Euphrates region namely the Sumerian, Babylonian and Chaldean empires contributed greatly to the building of the earliest pharmacopoeia of mankind. An Egyptian papyri dated from about 1,600 BC has survived to our day to reveal the ancient use of plant, animal and mineral concoctions, many of which are still in use.

The Chinese during the Yin dynasty of 1,500 BC recorded formulas for herbal preparations by inscription on prophet or oracle bones with over 160,000 being uncovered and cataloged by archeologists. Among those listed are coriander, fennel and thyme which were commonly used during that era for medicine and flavoring foods; minerals including iron, lime and magnesium; and products originating from animal sources such as honey, tallow and ox liver. The Hebrew Scriptures of the Holy Bible are rich in references to herbs commonly used at that time such as frankincense and myrrh, (at one time more costly than gold), cinnamon and mandrake. One herbal formula, Balm of Gillead has remained listed in pharmaceutical literature into our twentieth century.

Contributions from the middle east with the Ayurvedic medicine of India and outer lying medeopersian kingdoms soon became incorporated as a result of conquests and trading. As time passed the subsequent Greek and Roman Empires added their influence affecting the remaining cultures in the old world.

Use of Herbs in North America

ver 4,000 years ago, the first inhabitants of North America saw the wonders of the universe personified in the gifts of the earth, namely the healing power of herbs. Excavations of ancient archeological sites have unearthed many implements used by early man in North America specifically for the grinding and preparation of botanical medicines. Handed down from generation to generation by oral tradition, the sacred formulas used for childbirth, curing of disease and treating injuries were each tribe's manifestation of their place in the natural scheme of things. The prominent healers were the medicine men or shamans and medicine societies who interceded to assist the sick tribal member.

Native American medicine men and women were influenced by their dreams and taught that understanding of medicine came to them while in a trance or dream state. Using drums and rattles and the smoking of the "sacred" tobacco the shaman would enter into a semiconscious state by which he could "spirit travel" to the world of the supernaturals to seek the soul of the ailing person for a healing. Animal totems such as the coyote, eagle and bear were assigned to the four cardinal directions on the symbolic medicine wheel. Associated with four distinct personality types, diseases and root medicines, the eagle of the east represented the energies of wisdom and understanding whereas the coyote epitomized the powers of growth and compassion, attributes of the south.

The medicine pouch or bundle was used by many Native American tribal members whether shamans or not. Prepared from birth it often contained the person's umbilical stump wrapped and put aside by one's mother. It also contained sacred tobacco and perhaps a small carved animal totem or effigy thought to be the person's animal helper. Most young men went on a vision quest of isolation, fasting and prayer to seek just who this special helper would be.

Many tribes, specifically my Six Nations Iroquois Confederacy ancestors were a tribe who relied in part on agriculture. Drawings from the 1600's show elaborate encampments of elm bark covered longhouses encircled with groves and orchards of native fruit and nut trees. Outside of the longhouses or Iroquois family dwellings were the gardens which were the sole property of the woman as was the home and all of its belongings. Wild plants and edibles were at first "wild crafted" or gathered in the woods. Yet there is a legend,

"The Miracle of the Seeds" which speaks of three Iroquois maidens who left their homes to gather berries in the forest. Commonly, sunflower seeds were taken along in a buckskin pouch as a portable source of nutritious food. On that day one maiden dropped and lost her pouch in the woodlands. After searching for the lost pouch in vain, they returned home Upon visiting the woods the following summer on another excursion, the young women discovered the pouch, only now with beautiful sunflowers growing up out of it. It was from this point that the secret of the seeds and cultivation became revealed to the Iroquois people. After that, many wild plants were grown close to home affording greater accessibility for the gathering and preparation of herbal products. After about 15 years the camping ground was abandoned for a new, more fertile site within the tribal hunting grounds. Now it was easy to take seeds and cuttings to the new land for planting and starting anew without losing the herbs or the long acquired wisdom for their use.

Upon arrival of the settlers to our shores, we had in place an organized system of medicinal healing arts replete with knowledgeable, skilled practitioners. In fact Native American medicine men were able to show the pioneers safer methods of birth control, mending of broken bones, surgical technique and care of wounds. The settlers on their part were eager to learn how to use these native preparations as medical doctors were scarce in the new world. Hence "frontier medicine" emerged and was anxiously embraced by the common people although practitioners of orthodox medicine of the time rejected it. Frontiersmen living and trading among the natives began to document and publish books detailing the plant medicines commonly used by the North American tribes.

As early as 1672 John Josselyn wrote and published "New England's Rarities Discovered" which listed the medicinal uses of snakeroot, willow, slippery elm and sassafras as learned from the local tribes. By the time of George Washington's death, another individual, Samuel Thomson rebelled against the orthodox medical practices of the day which included the heavy use of mercury and leeches. He countered with a revival of herbal medicine and whereas he did not give due credit to the source of his enlightenment, it was clear that his roots were indeed firmly planted in the herbal tradition of Native American ethnobotany. Thomson adopted the secret healing therapies of the sweat lodge and the use of lobelia as well as other herbs taken from the indigenous materia medica. His discernment's actually reached back to Europe via

England through a successor namely Dr. Albert Isaiah Coffin, who set up a similar protocol of patent medicines and self-treatment preparations. Wooster Beech then followed in 1850 with his "eclectic" dogma. By 1864 the splintered groups founded by each of these forerunners joined to form the National Association of Medical Herbalists. It exists down to our present day as the National Institute of Medical Herbalists, the oldest professional body of specialist herbal practitioners in Europe. Back in America patent medicines were all the rage, being hawked by "snake oil" salesmen across the western United States. Many were based on safe and effective Native American herbal formulas and sported elaborate drawings of "Indian Maidens" on the label to add authenticity. The horrible fact is that until the Pure Food and Drug Act of 1906, these patent medicine bottlers did not have to disclose the content of the addictive substances they added to their product to assure repeat customers. Alcohol, opium, morphine, heroin and marijuana extracts were common additives even though they were known to cause drug addiction. The Pure Food and Drug Act required manufactures of patent medicines and drug products to, for the first time list the amount of alcohol and like adulterants right on the product label. The Shirley Amendment further modified this act in 1912 to prevent labels of patent medicines to contain "any statement...regarding the curative or therapeutic effect...which is fraudulent." At the turn of the century a then budding pharmaceutical manufacturer Eli Lilly and Company sought to patent an echinacea elixir for market. Under Teddy Roosevelt's administration, however, the patent was denied. The reason? One can not patent something that is already available to everyone for free. From that time until now herbs have been clearly defined as a product of public domain. Since herbs are not "patentable" products, pharmaceutical companies veered away from using botanicals in medicines although even as of 1996 up to 40% of all prescription drugs used in the United States are derived from plant or natural sources. Many herbs such as willow bark, which lead to the discovery of aspirin and Peruvian bark yielding quinine to treat dysentery were some of the numerous Native American herbal contributions that changed medical history and improved disease control the world over.

Native Healing Traditions Practiced Today

In our computer age of fast paced technology the usefulness of herbal healing alternatives is no longer relegated to the realm of "folk medicine". Scientific studies done in this country and abroad have given us perceptiveness as to the therapeutic action of numerous herbal formulas. Noteworthy is Merck and Company, a major pharmaceutical giant of the northeast, who recently purchased one square mile of tropical rainforest for the sole purpose of researching medical applications of the plethora of plant species represented there. Although it may seem like a very small area to study, one square mile of tropical rainforest has more biodiversity than the entire state of New York! Actually it would take a millennium to sift through the many uses of the herbs available there, so special scientists are enlisted to observe and document the native people's implementation of herbs gathered locally. Pharmacognocists or scientists who study medicines derived from plants and natural sources have the tedious task of separating myth from medicine in an effort to isolate the bioactive chemical in the plant that makes it so effective. Since herbs are highly complex, weeding through the 100 or more individual chemical constituents unique to the make-up of each plant often is a laborious endeavor. Complicating the problem even more is the reality that local native traditional healers are dying off without passing on this centuries acquired wisdom to younger progeny. Due to this fact there is a race for research before both they and the rainforests themselves vanish.

Here in North America, Native American tribes are struggling to maintain our unique culture. When I visited St. Regis Mohawk Reservation, (known to our people as Akwesasne) in upstate New York a few years ago I saw a fierce determination to remain independent in all aspects of life. This included the caring for one's self by natural and herbal means. I spent time with two of the midwives who "caught babies" on a regular basis on the reserve. What struck me was their confidence and ability to work with our native women assigning them the dignity and respect they deserved. Iroquois women are encouraged to be active in the birthing process, not passive. The midwives were involved in that course by making herbal medicine for both the mother and child during the stages of pregnancy and birth. A woman is therefore supported yet empowered. Tobacco is often burned outside of the birthing place and if there is a full moon, a ceremony may be performed complete with the making of full moon bread. Birth is truly a time for reflection as the baby is often named from an extraordinary event surrounding the birth.

The use of herbs today is not exclusively the domain of medicine men and midwives although they are still the teachers. The Native American concept of medicine is to enable the patient the ability to take part in caring for their bodies in a way that is in total harmony with nature. It is the handing down of this healing wisdom that enriches the lives of each passing generation.

CHAPTER TWO

The Medicine Pouch—Your Guide to Indigenous Herbs

hat is an herb? Well the answer depends upon whom you ask. To a botanist, an herb is a plant that meets specific criteria for growth and regeneration. For example, most of us envision herbs as plants which are pungent and fragrant but in actuality, herbs span the entire breadth of the plant kingdom. To native peoples, however, foods and herbs were used interchangeably for both medicine and nutrition. As you will see, most herbs are very life sustaining in their own right providing the body with essential vitamins, minerals and enzymes.

Traditional Native American healers are specialists in many disciplines. My great-grandmother was a midwife among the Eastern Band Cherokee and was respected for her profession. Midwives saw the woman from menarche, (first menstrual cycle) to menopause and offered herbal remedies specific for the changing phases of her life. Here it can be seen how the woman was revered as an individual as well as an important member of society. During the birthing process, women were empowered to actively participate in the birth even though sedating herbs were readily available. Instead, loving support and useful encouragement were the primary medicine given to her. A midwife could see reflected through the woman's eyes the miracle of birth, even as it had happened for her as a young mother. That bond between midwife and patient lasted a lifetime as she was often consulted during the postpartum period and beyond.

The shaman or medicine man is most often characterized by ritualistic chants and spiritism. However, the medicine man or woman more often than not had a working knowledge of the native botanicals at their disposal. You might think of the medicine man's modern day medical equivalent as being that of a psychiatrist. Convincing the patient that he could employ supernatural powers to help them called upon the effect of placebo. Isn't believing in your doctor 90% of the healing process? Likewise the medicine men appealed to the belief system of the person already in place. Through a bit of slight of hand, the medicine man would display the removal of diseased organs through "bloodless surgery", a visual confirmation that a cure had been affected. Observation of the mind's effect on the body's power to heal was made early on by native peoples and continues to be the subject of intense medical investigation today.

The Six Nation's Iroquois have secret medicine societies. Only those who really wish to help others are taught the traditional ways. According to one of the Eel clan mothers, Alice Papineau of the Onondaga, "We have drummers and singers in our medicine ceremonies. Nobody would ever know it because we don't allow non-Native people at all, because right away they go and write about it. And as I said, only people who have been afflicted by the sickness are invited to a ceremony." Not to be overlooked is the sense of community built into the healing rites. Physical human touch, singing, playing of music and dancing all come together to lift the spirits from the characteristic depression that often accompanies illness. Keep in mind also that our food is our medicine and our medicine, our food so there is a blurred distinction between the two. Even without traditional ceremony, anyone can benefit from the wisdom of Native American herbs for health and healing. Here are some of the most historically useful botanicals that should make up your own medicine pouch.

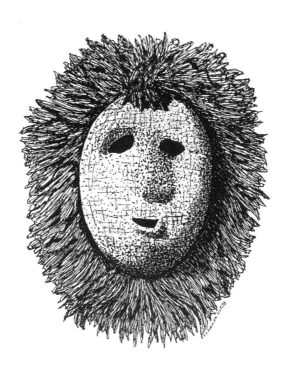

Beechnut *(Fagus grandifolia)* My Iroquois ancestors enjoyed beechnuts both roasted and raw in late fall after the first real frosts had caused them to drop from the trees. My people ground the inner bark of the beech tree into a fine flour for bread while the tender spring leaf shoots were prepared as delicious greens. Since about 20% of the nut consists of oil, this too was extracted and utilized for cooking and seasoning other dishes.

MEDICINAL ACTIONS: Both the bark and the leaves are astringent, tonic and antiseptic.

TRADITIONAL USES: Used by native peoples for stomach ulcers, kidney and bladder infections and dysentery.

MODERN MEDICINE: New research is showing this medicinal tree to be helpful in controlling Diabetes. The leaves produce a nerve calming substance which may be of benefit for nervous stomach disorders as well.

DOSAGE: 1 teaspoon of dried beech leaves in one cup of boiling water. Let steep 3-5 minutes. Therapeutic dose, 3-4 cups per day.

Beebalm *(Monarda didyma L.)* A prominent member of the mint family, my paternal Aunt Laura used to mention this herb to me as a child. It grows from New York to Georgia and as far west as Michigan along the banks of streams and among the underbrush.

MEDICINAL ACTIONS: Analgesic, diaphorhetic, (induces sweating) and verimifuge (expels intestinal worms)

TRADITIONAL USES : Used by many eastern woodland tribes for cold, flu, fever, bloating gas, stomach disorders, nosebleeds, sleeplessness heart problems and measles.

MODERN MEDICINE: Although the leaves have been used by physicians in the past to expel worms and alleviate flatulence, Beebalm is getting a second look as a safe and effective remedy for intestinal worms.

DOSAGE: Leaves of Beebalm must be boiled to extract medicinal properties. Make a decoction by boiling 1 tsp. of dried leaves to one pint of water for at least 5 minutes. This minty brew can be taken in the about of 3-4 cups per day.

Black Birch *(Betula lenta L.)* Both sweet and black birch have contributed to the development of one of the most widely used over the counter medications known to modern man...aspirin! Native Americans used the bark for fevers, coughs and stomach aches. From observation of the native uses of both the bark and twigs, it was seen that the essential oil distilled from the bark could relieve the pain of rheumatism, gout, neuralgia and arthritis. Similar to wintergreen in chemical composition and fragrance, birch's bioactive ingredient is methyl salicylate and was naturally derived by distillation in Appalachia up until around the turn of the century. Now methyl salicyclate is synthetically manufactured in pharmaceutical labs using menthol as the precursor.

MEDICINAL ACTIONS: Analgesic, anti-inflammatory. WARNING the essential oil is toxic and easily absorbed through the skin. Fatalities have been reported with the highly concentrated distilled oil, but not teas made from the bark or leaves.

TRADITIONAL USES: Birch twig tea was used by my people as a antipyretic or fever reliever. It was also appreciated for its ability to alleviate muscle pain often associated with fever. Native peoples would likewise use birch for kidney and bladder infections.

MODERN MEDICINE: Aspirin was originally isolated from Native American medicinal trees such as birch and willow. These barks contain salicylic acid, molecularly similar to acetyl salicylic acid, the chemical formula for aspirin. Today this over the counter drug is recommended for its blood thinning properties to help prevent platelet clots which may lead to a second heart attack.

DOSAGE: 1 ounce of fresh birch twigs can be made into an infusion by steeping for 3-5 minutes in a pint of boiling water. 2-3 cups per day.

Blue Cohosh *(Caulophyllum thalictroides, Mich.)* Common names include blue ginseng, papoose root and squaw root and for good reason. My family's women has used blue cohosh for everything from menstrual cramps to childbirth. I have personally used it to relieve the discomfort of childbirth to enjoy a nearly pain free homebirth experience. Being a oxytocic, it promotes the secretion of oxytocin, the "childbirth hormone" necessary for effective uterine contractions. A decoction of the root was given to babies for colicky cramps, hence the other common name, papoose root.

MEDICINAL PROPERTIES: Oxytocic, Dysmenorrhea, Parturient, Sedative, Antispasmodic.

TRADITIONAL USES: Native American women were encouraged to be active during childbirth, often walking and squatting the whole time. Blue cohosh has a mild sedating effect and speeds up a sluggish labor. Many tribal women went to a little hut on the edge of the encampment during their menstrual cycle where the blue cohosh root was given to them for relief of cramps. In fact "squaw" is derived from an Algonquin word for "women in their monthly blood flow".

MODERN MEDICINE: Rich in minerals, blue cohosh helps to alkalize the blood and urine. As early as 1925 Drs. Wood and Ruddock recorded blue cohosh as being "especially valuable in epileptic fits." They also noted its application in treating mouth sores and throat ulcerations in their patients. Rich in pH balancing minerals such as magnesium, potassium and calcium, blue cohosh can quickly alkalize overly acid blood and urine.

DOSAGE: For a spasmodic cough steep one ounce of the root in 1 pint of boiling water. Two tablespoons taken every three hours allows the blue cohosh to act like an expectorant. For an easy labor and childbirth, take one cup of infusion per day and only in the two weeks prior to birth. I've used it, it works!

Cattail *(Typha latifolia)* The characteristic brown hot-dog shaped female flowerheads make the cattail one of the most easily recognizable plants in our fresh marshes and pond areas. The fuzzy seed coverings from inside the mature flowerhead were used as pillow and mattress stuffing by early settlers.

MEDICINAL PROPERTIES: Anti-diarrheal, nephritic, (dissolves kidney stones)

TRADITIONAL USES: Native peoples would trek into the swampy marsh lands to harvest the edible rhizomes, shoots, anthers and pollen of the common cattail. A poultice was made of the roots, or, more accurately, rhizomes, which have a gelatin like consistency. This jelly-paste was then applied to sores, boils, inflammations, burns and scalds. Native mothers used the fluffy insides of the cattail as an absorbent "disposable" diaper material which also prevented chafing irritation common to infants. The tender, young flower tops were eaten for diarrhea while the root was used for both diarrhea and dysentery.

MODERN MEDICINE: Although this plant has been widely used for food by humans for thousands of years it is suspect of being toxic to free grazing animals. A related species of narrowleaf Cattail has been used to dissolve and expel kidney stones.

DOSAGE: 1 teaspoon of cattail rhizome placed in one pint of boiling water is the standard infusion or tea for this plant. 2-3 cups per day have been reported to help break up kidney stones, otherwise known as gravel.

Cherry, Wild (*Prunus Sertina*) Inhabits a wide range of dry woods from Nova Scotia to Florida and Texas to North Dakota. The fruits of the wild cherry turn blackish in color when ripe and are sweet with a tart aftertaste.

MEDICINAL PROPERTIES: Sedatives, expectorant

TRADITIONAL USES: The fragrant inner bark was used by native peoples to prepare a syrup mixed with maple for coughs, colds, fevers, pneumonia, bronchitis and other lung ailments.

MODERN MEDICINE: Wild cherry bark still holds a place in the United States Pharmacopoeia as an active ingredient in cough syrups such as Cheracol.

DOSAGE: WARNING Non-fruit parts of the tree such as the inner bark, leaves and seeds contain a cyanide like substance, prunasin, which is converted to a very toxic hydrocyanic acid in the digestive tract. Nonetheless, it is still listed in the U.S. Pharmacopoeia.

Corn (*Zea mays*) This truly identifiable Native American food crop was actually exported to Ireland during the great potato famine to relieve the starvation of the mid 1800's. Considered more a food than a medicine, native peoples enjoyed a variety of products from the many varieties of corn which they cultivated.

MEDICINAL PROPERTIES: Diuretic, hypoglycemic and hypotensive agent

TRADITIONAL USES: Corn silk is well documented as a safe and effective diuretic for cystitis, gout and rheumatism. Native peoples make a tea of corn silk for these purposes. Ground cornmeal was made into a paste base for herbal poultices and applied to the skin. A most valuable food crop, it has its place in many of our traditional foods and medicines. In fact, no part of the corn plant went to waste. In the summer, the dried corn husks from the previous fall were woven into airy moccasins, faceless dolls, mats and ceremonial masks.

MODERN MEDICINE: Corn oil has been followed by the health sciences for arteriosclerosis and hyperlipidemia, or high cholesterol. The corn seed or kernels contain allantoin, a wound healing substance which also accelerates cellular turnover in the skin. Corn silk has been studied and proven effective as a diuretic in animal trials. Additionally, these same types of studies using animals have held up showing corn extract to be helpful in lowering blood sugar and blood pressure.

Dock, Yellow or Curly *(Rumex crispus)* So named yellow dock because in the months June through September, the roots are yellowish when sliced in half to reveal its cross section.

MEDICINAL PROPERTIES: Laxative/ anti-diarrheal depending on the concentration taken. Alternative, astringent, tonic and antiscorbutic.

TRADITIONAL USES: Indigenous tribes collected yellow dock leaves early in the spring while still tender and prepared them much the same way people eat kale or spinach today. In fact, it is often called wild spinach for this reason. The roots were pulled up and made into a decoction to be used for the internal and external treatment of skin sores, rheumatism and sore throat. Enlarged lymph glands and liver ailments have also been indications for the use of dried yellow dock root as it was thought to purify "bad blood."

MODERN MEDICINE: Pharmacologists have isolated the presence of both anthraquionones which produce a laxative action and tannins which can safely arrest diarrhea as both being present in yellow dock. Anthraquionones additionally have been seen to inhibit and arrest the spread of ringworm which is actually an aggressive fungus as well as contagious fungi. Tannins are currently being studied for their antioxidant properties and their ability to limit free radical damage due to the natural oxidation of tissue cells. Yellow dock is very rich in minerals, especially a quite absorbable form of organic iron.

DOSAGE: 1 teaspoon of ground root to one cup of boiling water steeped for 2-3 minutes. The longer it steeps, the more tannins or anti-diahrreal properties will be extracted. For use as a laxative, steep for only a minute or so to leave the tannins intact. Standard dose is 2-3 cups per day for therapeutic use. Dock has a characteristically bitter taste so you might wish to make a syrup by boiling 1/2 pound of the crushed root in one pint of natural syrup. In this case, one teaspoon 2-3 times per day is recommended. bruised or crushed fresh dock leaves can be extremely applied as a poultice to remove skin ulcers, tumors and skin eruptions.

Echinacea *(e. angustifolia)* Commonly known as purple coneflower, Echinacea was perhaps the most widely known herb known to the prairie tribes west of what is today called Ohio. So named "the sacred herb" by many plains tribes, it was used for everything from snakebite to typhoid fever. Many tribes recognized its value as a natural antiseptic.

MEDICINAL PROPERTIES: Antiseptic, immunostimulant. It induces the lymphatic system to clear away wastes and toxins. Moreover, it has a definite antibacterial activity.

TRADITIONAL USES: The Dakota Sioux used the raw scraped root of Echinacea, considered the therapeutic part of the plant, to treat rabies, infected wounds and as a remedy for snakebite. Taken internally and used as a poultice externally, Echinacea root has a long standing history of being one of the most efficacious remedies known to the first Americans.

MODERN MEDICINE: Modern clinical studies show Echinacea's ability to increase properdin levels, a plasma protein which is part of the non-specific immune system. Due to this activity, it helps the white blood cells to surround and destroy foreign bacteria and viruses. The newest research is showing Echinacea to be helpful in lessening the incidence of the common cold and flu.

DOSAGE: Steep 1 teaspoon of ground Echinacea root in a cup of boiling water for 1/2 an hour. No need to boil as in preparing a decoction. Strain off the plant material and take 1 tablespoon 3-4 times per day for therapeutic effect. For prophalasis or to help prevent infections, one cup of Echinacea tea per day for 4-6 weeks, then stopping for two weeks is often recommended. This is called cycling. You are simply trying to nudge your immune system's response, so it is not necessary to take Echinacea everyday. WARNING: Individuals with auto-immune system disorders should not use Echinacea.

Elderberry *(Sambucus canadenis, L.)* All parts of this plant yielded medicine to early native peoples. The flowers, berries, leaves and inner bark were noted for their healing properties. Used in a poultice to stop bleeding, the Elderberry bark could also prevent severe bruising which often were the lot of the Iroquois warriors both from battle or lively games of Lacrosse.

MEDICINAL PROPERTIES: Diuretic, laxative and emetic. A mild diaphoretic, stimulant and carminative.

TRADITIONAL USES: Mixed with peppermint, Elderberry leaves would be used for colds, to bring out a sweat and induce vomiting. Many Native American remedies were revered for just these last two effects, as sweating and emesis (vomiting) were ways to quickly and effectively remove poisons from the system.

MODERN MEDICINE: Elderberry elixir is now being investigated for its ability to combat many cold viruses responsible for colds and the flu.

DOSAGE: WARNING: Unripe Elderberries, bark, and leaves contain cyanide and can cause poisoning and severe diarrhea. Cooked fruits can be safely used, however. Elderberry elixir can be made, (see section on making your own herbal products,) and mixed into water. General dosage is 1 tablespoon of elixir to 1 cup of water.

Goldenseal *(Hydrastis canadensis)* Actually a member of the buttercup family, this beneficial plant is quickly becoming scarce in its native habitat ranging from Vermont to Georgia. This is because over-collection in the Eastern deciduous forests is making this herb increasingly rare.

MEDICINAL PROPERTIES: Antibacterial, sedative, anti-convulsant

TRADITIONAL USES: Goldenseal is considered synergistic with Echinacea. The medicinal portion of the plant most valued is the root. Native peoples made a decoction or tincture and used it as a gargle for throat infections, pharyngitis and bronchitis. A weak tea wash was traditionally used for eye infections and irritations of the digestive system and uterus.

MODERN MEDICINE: Its sedative properties have been demonstrated experimentally to lower blood pressure . Goldenseal root has been found to contain berberine, a germ killing substance which also acts to control seizures and encourages bile secretion to help in the breakdown of dietary fats. Recently, studies have disproved the myth that the use of Goldenseal will mask the presence of morphine in drug urine tests.

DOSAGE: WARNING: Should not be used during pregnancy. An external eyewash can be made by boiling the Goldenseal roots for 5-7 minutes. Tinctures, (alcohol based) can also be made but should be avoided for use in soothing mucus membranes as the alcohol can be too irritating. Combined in a salve with Echinacea, it makes an effective topical treatment for almost any skin disorder.

False and Solomon's Seal (*Polygonatum biflorum*) This plant's range is from Connecticut to Florida and as far West as Nebraska. This plant has a wide range of uses by native peoples due to its many medicinal properties.

MEDICINAL PROPERTIES: Anti-inflammatory, carminative, antiseptic and laxative

TRADITIONAL USES: Native Americans appreciated the laxative effect of Solomon's Seal to ease indigestion, constipation and the hemorrhoids that often follow. The roots were prepared into an antiseptic wash which was applied to all types of skin infections and irritations. Respiratory ailments, coughs and colds were treated with this plant as well as menorrhagia or profuse bleeding and insomnia.

DOSAGE: Fresh root can be made by grinding the roots into a poultice and then applying directly to the affected area. A decoction of root tea can be made by using 1 teaspoon of powdered root to one pint of boiling water. If whole, allow the root to boil for 5-7 minutes. 1 cup per day can be used constitutionally for rheumatism and to encourage restful sleep.

Hydrangea *(Hydrangea arborescens)* Commonly known as "seven barks" due to the difference in color variations of the cross section of the inner barks. The root of this widely distributed deciduous tree is considered the most potent medicinal part.

MEDICINAL PROPERTIES: Diuretic, nephritic, cathartic

TRADITIONAL USES: Used by native peoples to ease the excruciatingly painful passing of kidney stones and gravel. Obviously this would consistently qualify hydrangea as a kidney and urinary tract tonic. Quite interestingly, Hydrangea is also indicated for rheumatism, which is thought to run parallel to excessive calcium deposits and high body fluid alkalinity.

MODERN MEDICINE-Experimentally, large doses of Hydrangea root have been shown to cause stomach upset and bloody diarrhea although traditionally native peoples chewed the bark for stomach complaints and heart trouble.

DOSAGE: Due to the potential problem as described above, hydrangea root should not be taken internally. It can, however be prepared by scraping the fresh bark and applying it externally as a poultice for burns, sprains, tumors and sore muscles.

Juniper (*Juniperus communis*) Juniper is related to the pine family of evergreens. All parts of the shrub are used for medicine. French country folk would make an antiseptic juniper tar out of the inner wood of the branches and trunk.

MEDICINAL PROPERTIES: Diuretic, carminative, urinary antiseptic and laxative. Considered toxic if used in large amounts or frequently.

TRADITIONAL USES: Native people used juniper externally for snakebite, cancers, sore aching muscles, arthritis and rheumatism. Internally the berries were used in a limited way for worms, stomach ulcers, respiratory aliments, colds and constipation.

MODERN MEDICINE: Juniper berries are used commercially today to flavor alcoholic beverages such as gin but are also included in many laxative preparations. Its primary action is that of a diuretic yet it found its way in both the U.S. Pharmacopoeia and the National Formulary for several years as a treatment for suppressed menstruation.

DOSAGE: About 10-15 small juniper berries can be mashed with a fork to break the skin. Pour 1 pint of boiling water over them and let steep for 20-30 minutes. Juniper berry tincture is also a very convenient way to make a tea. In this case 1 teaspoon of tincture can be added to boiling water for a quick infusion.

Jerusalem Artichoke

(*Helianus tuberosus*) A member of the sunflower family which is also an indigenous plant. The leaf, stalk and flowers were made into an infusion to treat rheumatism and arthritic complaints. The roots or tubers of the plant were roasted with nut butter and served in a way that many today enjoy baked potatoes.

MEDICINAL PROPERTIES:
Anti-inflammatory and analgesic.

TRADITIONAL USES: The flowers were often eaten fresh to provide relief for rheumatic joint complaints. The tuberous roots of the plant were dug, rinsed in spring water and rubbed with seed oils before roasting. Nut butters of beech, hickory and sunflower were then added to the Jerusalem Artichoke for extra flavor and nutrition.

MODERN MEDICINE: Scientists have isolated inulin, a polysaccharide, which may help to control diabetes present in Jerusalem Artichoke.

DOSAGE: A tea of the stalks and leaves can be made with 1 teaspoon of dried plant to 1 cup of boiling water. Let this infusion steep for 3-5 minutes. Traditionally used for rheumatism, this tea can be taken in amounts of 2-3 cups per day therapeutically. The tubers of the Jerusalem Artichoke are very nutritious and easily digestible. You can dig your own roots of the plant and prepare them with a little almond oil before roasting them in a 350 degree oven until done in the center. Other companies such as Deboles have made wonderful pasta products from Jerusalem Artichoke for years. Look for them in your local health food store.

Maple *(Acer-rubrum)* Commonly called the sugar maple, this abundant and useful tree is found from the north woods of Maine and as far west as Michigan. Maple syrup is made by boiling down the sap of the tapped trees in spring. Native American tribes were documented as doing this when the first settlers arrived on our shores. This was not a lazy person's task. It takes about 40 gallons of sap to boil down into 1 gallon of syrup. One big Maple will yield about 5-6 lbs. of sap per season.

MEDICINAL PROPERTIES: Tonic, astringent, diuretic

TRADITIONAL USES: Maple seeds are edible after removing the "propellers" and many native people enjoyed them roasted. Also the inner bark was ground into a fine flour and made into bread. Its astringent properties were utilized to the full as a tonic for sore, irritated eyes, a common complaint of dwellers of homes with fire pits for cooking. The syrup was given to women who had just given birth to help them regain the strength in their muscles they had prior to paturation. The primary confection of the northern eastern woodlands was maple syrup. It was used to sweeten and add taste variety to corn meal porridge, soups, vegetables and fruits.

MODERN MEDICINE: Maple syrup is rich in natural enzymes, vitamins and minerals. Highly nutritious, it is a wonderful alternative to sucrose or white table sugar which contains no vitamins and conversely causes spikes in blood sugar.

DOSAGE: Maple syrup can be used in an infusion of one tablespoon to 1 pint of boiling water. 3-4 cups per day of this maple tea is considered therapeutic.

Mint *(Menthia piperita)* Although this genus has origins in Eurasia and Australia, it has come to be embraced by native American people for its many applications. Spearmint, wintergreen and meadowsweet are all mints with similar properties. Peppermint is the familiar flavor in chewing gum and other confections as well as toothpaste and mouthwash. As a child I can remember going to the nurse's office and being given essential oil of peppermint in a little cup of water for a stomach ache. It did work well!

MEDICINAL PROPERTIES: Stomachic, Stimulant, carminative and analgesic in large amounts.

TRADITIONAL USES: My paternal

Aunt Laura would send us off in the morning with a hot cup of peppermint tea. She told me that her grandmother, a Cherokee midwife, used Bee Balm, also in the mint family, in the same way, to prepare the stomach for the first meal of the day by stimulating digestion. Mint leaves were usually gathered at the end of summer when they have the highest amount of volatile oil present. For colds and the flu, mint was used to help quell the accompanying nausea, vomiting, body ache and fever.

MODERN MEDICINE: Pharmacognocists have isolated a specific compound in mint called salicylic acid. Similar to acetyl salicylic acid, the chemical name for aspirin, it is an effective analgesic, antipyretic and stimulant. In fact the use of peppermint has been seen to strengthen heart muscles and cleanse the entire system.

DOSAGE: Although mint is generally safe to use, people who are allergic to aspirin should not take any kind of mint. Likewise pennyroyal mint is considered poisonous and should be avoided by all, especially pregnant women in whom this herb has been shown to produce miscarriage. If you are on blood thinners such as Coumadin, mint should not be used as it will prolong prothrombin times leading to excessive bleeding. The usual infusion of one ounce of herb to one cup of boiling water steeped for 3-5 minutes is recommended for constitutional use. For therapeutic use, up to 3 cups per day can be taken.

Nettle *(Urtica dioca)* Commonly known as stinging nettles this plant can be found throughout the U.S. and Canada. It is so named because of the stinging hairs along the stem which prick the skin and irritate it by emitting a bitter, pain inducing fluid.

MEDICINAL PROPERTIES: Diuretic, astringent

TRADITIONAL USE: Native peoples used stalks of nettle to combat the discomfort of skin irritations. More importantly it was given by native midwives during pregnancy and after paturation as an excellent "blood" builder. Nettle, rich in absorbable organic iron, acted as insurance against post partum hemorrhage and to promote a copious milk supply. Poultices made of crushed leaves were applied to the site of an injury to arrest profuse bleeding and soothe rheumatic joints. It also works well as a diuretic assisting in arthritic and rheumatic complaints.

MODERN MEDICINE: Recent clinical study has shown nettle to act on white blood cells assisting the coagulation process and facilitating the formation of hemoglobin in red blood cells. Its CNS or sedative abilities have been shown by its action in inhibiting the stressful effects of adrenaline. Rich in vitamins C, B-complex and trace mineral salts, nettles contain glucokinins, a substance responsible for its anti-diabetic activity. The acrid substance in the aforementioned stinging hairs contain several amines, namely histamine, serotonin and choline making it useful in balancing the brain's neurotransmitters.

DOSAGE: 1 oz of finely chopped dried herb is steeped in 1 pint of water for 3-5 minutes. As a diuretic, several cups can be taken throughout the day.

Plantain (*Plantago major*) A weed known by native tribes as "white man's foot" because it seemed to spring up everywhere the settlers went! Obviously not native to North America, it was heartily embraced for its healing properties.

MEDICINAL PROPERTIES: Antiseptic, diuretic, astringent

TRADITIONAL USES: Native peoples quickly saw this weed spread across the continent, carried by invading settlers and their livestock. Taking advantage of its proliferation, the leaves were bruised and applied to wounds as an antiseptic poultice.

MODERN MEDICINE: A confirmed anti-microbial, plantain's use as an antiseptic wound dressing has been confirmed.

DOSAGE: Fresh leaves can serve as a soothing bandage if you're injured out in the field. In fact, a wonderful healing salve can be made of plantain alone or combined with other herbs.

Red Clover *(Trifolium pratense)* Although true clovers are said to have originated in south-western Asia and southeastern Europe, there are more than eighty species identified as indigenous to North America.

MEDICINAL PROPERTIES: Sedative, alterative

TRADITIONAL USES: Both the blossoms and leaves have been used for malignant cancers, kidney problems and even whooping cough for which native American tribes had no immunity. A pleasant tasting tea made from the blossoms was calming and helped to induce sleep. Native women used it also during menopause to help balance hormonal fluctuations.

MODERN MEDICINE: Clover is naturally rich in trace minerals and earth salts present in a balanced, absorbable form. The leaves have been studied and the traditional use of clover leaf has been validated as the leaves do contain isoflavonoids, namely plant estrogens. Although weak, they will interact with a woman's estrogen receptors enough to effect an increased production of natural estrogen.

DOSAGE: A delicious and nutritious calming tea can be made with one ounce of clover blossoms to 1 pint of boiling water steeped for 3-5 minutes. For estrogen production the leaves should be used exclusively. Steep once ounce of clover leaves in one pint of water for 3-5 minutes for this application.

Red Raspberry *(Rubus idaeus)* Perhaps the most widely used plant by Native American midwives, both the fruits and leaves are rich in vitamins and minerals. Raspberries, like blackberries are not true berries, but clumps of drupelets massed together.

MEDICINAL PROPERTIES: Astringent, tonic, stimulant

TRADITIONAL USES: Native American midwives cared for women throughout their reproductive cycle. Red raspberry leaves were used to quell menstrual cramps, aid in the prevention of miscarriage, assure an easy labor and prevent post partum hemorrhage. Gathered as both food and medicine, the whole raspberry plant was part of every woman's medicine pouch.

MODERN MEDICINE: Chemical analysis has shown red

raspberries to be rich in a variety of absorbable vitamins and minerals. Also present is a substance called fragrine, an alkaloid present in the leaves which tones the muscles of the pelvic region including but not limited to the uterus. This would validate the traditional use of this plant for an easy labor.

DOSAGE: One ounce of raspberry leaves, (this may include some of the dried fruits) to one pint of water, steeped for 3-5 minutes will give you a standard infusion. For an easy labor, drink one cup once daily during the third trimester or last three months of the pregnancy. Raspberry leaf tea can also carry over into the post partum period as it is an excellent galactogogue that will encourage the production of high quality breastmilk. (See the formulas for Pregnancy and Breastfeeding Teas).

Sage *(Saliva officinalis)* Although not native to North American soils, sage has taken a prominent place in tribal medicine. Interestingly enough, before it was introduced to our soils the Chinese traded up to two cases of their tea for the English sage tea.

MEDICINAL PROPERTIES: Carminitive, antispasmodic, antiseptic and astringent.

TRADITIONAL USES: Native peoples use sage smudges which are made by burning dried sage and rubbing the ashes on the patient or area to be disinfected. A strong tea is made as a rinse for the hair and used especially by the women to add a deep shine and luster to black hair.

MODERN MEDICINE: Science is investigating sage's ability to lower blood sugar levels and promote bile flow. It has a mildly sedative effect and relaxes peripheral blood vessels.

DOSAGE: WARNING, sage should be avoided by pregnant and nursing women as it will dry up breast milk. Also avoid if you suffer from epileptic seizures as sage contains thujone, which can trigger such fits. Small amounts in cooking are very safe, however. For a wonder hair rinse for dark to black hair, prepare an infusion of 1 ounce of herb to 1 pint of water and steep for 10 minutes. This rinse alone or in combination with other herbs is very effective in relieving dandruff and restoring color to graying hair.

Willow Bark *(Salix alba)* Willow acts in a very similar way as quinine. Like quinine it is an astringent and a bitter digestive tonic useful in controlling low grade fevers. Willow offers analgesic properties and was documented by French chemist Leroux in the 19th century. He isolated an active chemical in willow and called it "salicine". By 1852 this substance was copied synthetically and by 1899 acetylsalicylic acid made its way to be marketed as aspirin.

MEDICINAL PROPERTIES: Astringent, analgesic, antipyretic.

TRADITIONAL USES: Even though it is difficult to trace when willow bark was first used as a fever reducer and pain reliever by American Indians, there are many notations that this was what was given during such times of illness. For rheumatism, Native peoples used the willow bark as an analgesic or pain reliever to ease stiffness. To arrest post partum hemorrhage, a very warm douche of willow bark was made and used by native midwives.

MODERN MEDICINE: Chemical isolates of willow are called salicylic acids and are found in many other plants such as wintergreen meadowsweet. Today acetyl salicylic acid, otherwise known as aspirin, offers anti-inflammatory and analgesic activities. Its use in the US alone is more than 35 million pounds!

DOSAGE: Like most barks, willow must be decocted or boiled in order to extract the medicinal properties from the tough, ligneous fibers. Being an astringent, it is very bitter to taste so you may wish to put the ground bark into gelatin capsules for administration. Willow bark applied topically as a poultice works well on sores and abscesses of all types.

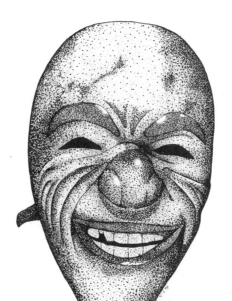

Growing Your Own Native Herbs

Herbs are basically "weeds" and will usually do well in poor soils that other plants would not thrive in. Among my father's people, the Cherokee, the herbs were planted and harvested during specific cycles of the moon. A growing moon or new moon was for planting. Even today many who grow their own herbs follow this ancient tradition recognizing that phases of the moon may have an effect on the growth and healing potential of the plant.

Herb seedlings can be started indoors in pots to grace a sunny kitchen window sill or planted outdoors in an herb garden setting. In either case you will quickly find yourself spoiled to having fresh, fragrant herbs at hand for use in making your herbal products and cooking.

A good place to find herbs is at your local nursery. Purchase young, healthy plants and transplant them outside after the last frost date for your region. For more variety you can purchase your seeds or seedlings from a nursery catalog which will carry a wider selection of herbs. (See Resource Section in the back of the book)

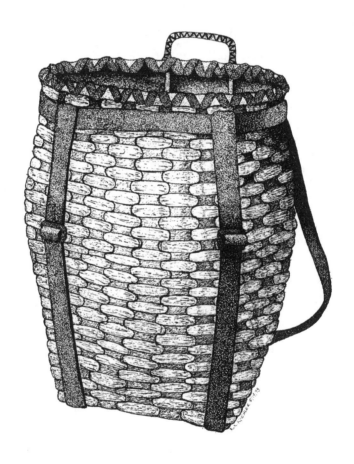

Harvesting and Drying

A general rule of thumb in harvesting your herbs is that one should pick early in the season for a light herbal product or when tender shoots are preferred and late August if the full compliment of essential oils and plant constituents is required. Certainly if you are wildcrafting or gathering a small amount of the plant leaves while leaving the main plant intact, you can pick anytime during the growing season. All the same, the more potent brews are generally made from herbs that have grown to maturity.

Many native peoples simply braided the stalks of their favorite herbs and hung them high in the rafters of their homes. The Iroquois longhouse could be seen strung with dried pumpkin, corn, beans, herbs and other foods for the winter. The heat rising from the individual family's cooking fires would slowly dry and preserve these food stores. You can do the same by tying the stems of your herbs into bundles and placing them upside down in a paper bag. Put the bag of herbs on a high kitchen cabinet shelf. Likewise to olden times, the heat from your cooking with slowly dry your herbs. This method takes about 2-3 weeks depending on outside humidity. This is why the dryer climate of the fall is so ideal for this method of preservation.

Framing Out Your Garden

Your herb garden can be as simple as a few pots on your windowsill or patio to a more elaborate formation in your garden. If growing indoors, the herbs will always be at the ready for use in teas and other herb products. Similarly, herbs grown on a sunny back porch in large pots offers the same convenience close at hand. As

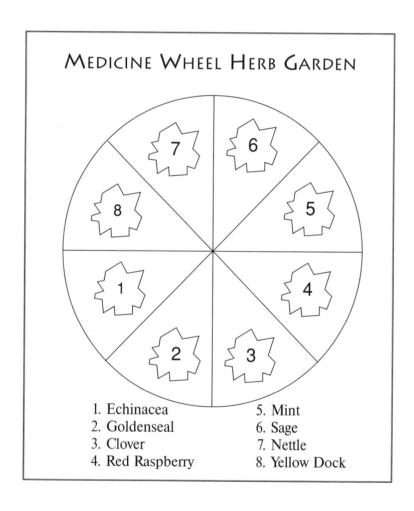

MEDICINE WHEEL HERB GARDEN

1. Echinacea
2. Goldenseal
3. Clover
4. Red Raspberry
5. Mint
6. Sage
7. Nettle
8. Yellow Dock

your plants grow in, trim off a few leaves for use as needed. As with most herbs, the more you cut, the more they will grow!

If you opt for traditional backyard herbal garden, you can plant in a "medicine wheel" pattern and have your herbs outwards from the "spokes", as can be seen on the previous page..

TRADITIONAL GARDEN PATCH

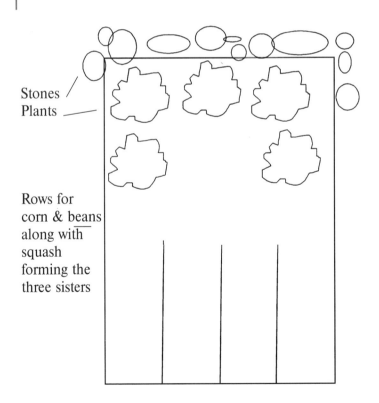

Stones
Plants

Rows for corn & beans along with squash forming the three sisters

If you already have an established vegetable garden, the addition of herbs around the borders will add interest, variety and the added benefit of protection of your garden produce from insects. Many herbs such as clover will actually enrich the soil, so you should plan to use it as ground cover for a season or two in a part of the garden that you would like to rest and reestablish.

Herbal Planting Chart:

Beebalm Perennial. Grows 3 to 4 feet tall. Plants threats: Aphids.

> NOTE: Likes full sun. Do not plants near any kind of mint. Works well to attract hummingbirds. Other common names: Indian nettle, Oswego tea and Bergamot.

Dock Perennial. Grows 1 to 4 feet tall.

> NOTE: Thrives in sun or shade. Keep confined to a small patch area to prevent it from taking over the rest of your garden. Other common names: Yellow dock.

Mint Perennial. Grows up to 30 inches. Plant threats: Aphids.

> NOTE: Grows best in well drained soil. To help control plants from taking over your garden, plant inside of small, bottomless flower pots and dig below top soil level. Other common names: There are hundreds of species of mint. Commonly found ones include, black mint, peppermint, spearmint, etc.

Nettle Perennial. Grows 2 to 6 feet tall.

> NOTE: Grows best in irrigated soil. Pretty immune to pests and diseases. Other common names: Common nettle and Stinging nettle.

New Jersey Tea Deciduous bush. Grows 2 to 3 feet tall.

> NOTE: Full sun or shade. Like Nettle it is pretty immune to pests and diseases. Other common names: Mountain sweet and Redroot.

Passionflower Climbing Plant. Grows up to 30 feet. Plant threats: Aphids, threes.

NOTE: Grows best in well drained and irrigated soil. Do not plant along side other pest and disease susceptible plants. Other common names: Apricot vine, Water lemon and Maypop.

Red Clover Perennial. Grows 1 to 2 feet.

NOTE: Full sun to partial shade. Quite immune to pests and disease. Works well to renew and rest soil of vegetable gardens. Other common names: Purple clover, Sweet clove and Trifolium.

Sage Perennial. Grows 1 to 2 feet tall.

NOTE: Grows in various soil conditions. Very immune to pests and diseases.

Other common names: Meadow sage, Spanish sage and Greek sage.

Soapwort Perennial. Grows 1 to 2 feet.

NOTE: Grows in various soil condition. Very immune to pests and diseases.

Other common names: Bouncing bet.

Planting Your Garden:

Frost dates are as important for herbs as they are for vegetables. You can get a jump on the growing season with your herbs, however, by growing them indoors. By the time you transfer them out, if you so decide, they will be large enough to fen for themselves. My father's people, the Eastern Band Cherokee were agriculturists, farming the rich soil of the southeastern Virginia. They believed in planting their fields and gardening on the new or growing "grandmother" moon. Scientists are investigating the effects of the moon's phases on the ocean's tide and farm crops. Try it! Perhaps there is something to this practice after all.

The idea of using the fish emulsion as fertilizer was known to Native American peoples especially of New England coastal states. Back then a fresh fish head was thrown in the seed mound and covered over. As it decomposed, it added valuable nitrogen and other needed elements to the soil as well as heat for optimal seed germination. The Iroquois still plant the Three Sisters, corn, beans and squash together. The corn stalk serves as a natural trellis for the climbing beans and squash. They are called the Three Sisters because eating this combination of complimentary amino acids can sustain life, as they come together to make a complete protein.

Maintaining Your Garden:

Native peoples realized that all life plays a part in maintaining a harmonious earth. Likewise in planting our gardens we realized that even weeds can contribute to the plot's overall health. For example, clover actually a legume, is one of our most nutritious herbs and enriches the soil by fixing nitrogen into it. Let clover and/or alfalfa grow over your fallow areas when you are giving the earth a rest and next season when you replant, the soil will be replenished. Weeds actually help prevent soil erosion with their strong root systems so I wouldn't recommend completely removing them.

Planting strong smelling herbs such as peppermint along the border of your garden will naturally repel insects and even many animal pests. If you plant Queen Anne's Lace and golden rod, they will attract beneficial wasps which enjoy these plant's abundant nectar. These wasps in turn have a voracious appetite for damaging aphids. Marigold flowers work in the same way to keep damaging insects at bay without resorting to chemical insecticides which can contaminate your crops. Another good idea is to use raised beds which are never walked upon which helps to keep the soil loose and uncompressed. Lawn clippings piled thick around the base of your plants will slowly nourish them and work to keep weeds down too.

CHAPTER THREE

MAKING YOUR OWN HERBAL FORMULAS

Overview of Herbal Remedy Preparation

This section combines the best of both the old and new world herbs. While respecting the native traditions in healing technique, other herbs have been included which are not indigenous to North America. These herbs nonetheless have been embraced and incorporated into time honored formulas to make them current for modern times.

Making your own herbal products at home is economical and quite aesthetically rewarding. Not only do you get to choose from the finest natural ingredients but you can vary the amounts to suit your own personal tastes and needs. You will also enjoy peace of mind that with every personal care product you make, you are replacing a commercial formula which often contains harmful chemicals, dyes and perfumes. Before you begin however, you might wish to have the following items on hand:

Wire Mesh Sieve	Cheesecloth
Tea Ball	Metal/glass funnel
Pyrex Glass Cookware	Small glass jars
Mortar and pestle	Amber Bottles
	Cobalt blue bottles

A fine wire mesh sieve will be needed for straining herbal materials out of your products. Inert, (non-reacting) glass pots such as Pyrex are preferable to iron or aluminum which may react with the minerals and acids present in the herbs. Pyrex or heat tempered glass doesn't impart unwanted metallic by-products to your formulas and will heat uniformly, hence their established use in chemistry labs is well earned. Bulk herbs are almost always less expensive than tea bags and herb capsules. You can save a lot of money using the bulk herbs that you either have grown or purchased, but you'll need a tea ball to do this. A tea ball can be purchased at any supermarket or health food store and is simply a screwable metal ball with holes so that you can place your herbs inside. After filling the tea ball, it is then placed in a pot of hot water to steep or can even be boiled as in a decoction. This useful item will keep most of the plant material out of your finished product. Cheesecloth is used to keep small bits of leaves out of your product and is the outer covering for an herbal poultice. Tea bags, likewise, may be used for this application as a quick and simple topical poultice. A mortar and pestle can be purchased at most any store which specializes in cooking supplies. With it you can grind barks, roots, stems and seeds to a powdery fineness. Grinding exposes more of the surface area of the herb material to processing, making for a more complete extraction of the medicinal components.

Metal or glass funnels are wonderful for transferring hot or cold extracts or infusions into smaller necked bottles. Small amber storage bottles come in a range of sizes from one to several ounces. Iron oxide is added to glass which is naturally aqua colored and provides a good measure of UV or ultraviolet light protection. Cobalt blue bottles likewise come in a variety of sizes and offer protection from the deteriorating rays of the sun. In this case the element cobalt is added during the glass making process to impart its characteristic deep blue color.

Basic Herbal Products

Infusions

> 1 oz dried herb including flowers and leaves (about 2 1/2 oz. of fresh)
>
> 1 pint of freshly drawn boiling water
>
> Infusions are well suited for steeping the more tender flowers, leaves, fruits and buds or many herbs. Bring your water to a whistling boil and pour over herbs. Let steep for 5-10 minutes, understanding that the longer it steeps, the more bitter tasting tannins will be extracted. Here a tea ball for loose bulk tea is indispensable. Always use freshly drawn water. Using re-boiled or re-heated water will leave your infusion flat tasting due to all of the oxygen being used up.
>
> *Standard dosage:* 1/2 cup or 4ozs three times daily

Decoctions

> 1 ounce dried or 2 oz. of fresh herbal twigs, roots, stems, or barks
>
> 2 pints of cool water, (your end product will be reduced to 1 pint amount)
>
> Decoctions are well suited for extracting the medicinal properties of the pithy parts of the plant even including some berries. Some roots and barks require simmering of up to an hour to decoct out the desired plant material. Place your herb material in a Pyrex pot with 2 pints of cool water. Let simmer until the liquid is

reduced to about 1 pint. Strain off into a serving container or teacup.

Standard Dose: 1/2 cup three times daily.

Syrups

1 cup of fresh infusion or decoction

1 cup of honey, raw sugar or maple syrup

Heat one cup of your standard infusion or decoction of choice while adding one cup of honey, raw sugar or maple syrup. Keep stirring to fully dissolve all sugars. Cool down the mixture and pour into dark amber bottles for storage. The honey acts as a great, natural preservative while hiding the taste of some of the more unpalatable herbs.

Standard dosage: 5mls (equals about 1 teaspoon) three times a day.

Tinctures and Vinegars

1 oz dried herbs or 2 oz. fresh

1 pint of 80 proof, (40%) grain alcohol such as Vodka or Brandy

OR

1 pint of Apple cider vinegar

Wide mouth jar with sealable lid

Using a sterile wide mouth jar, pour the grain alcohol over the herbs. Store in a cool dark place and shake daily for two weeks. Strain off plant material and pour into dark amber bottles with eyedroppers. For a vinegar, prepare the same way as a tincture but replace the alcohol constituent with hot vinegar. Shake the mixture daily for 1 week then strain off plant material and dispense into amber dropper bottles.

Standard dosage: 20 drops under the tongue or 1 teaspoon three times per day.

Infused oils and Ointments

2 oz. dried herb or 3oz of fresh

1 cup of cold pressed almond or sunflower seed oil

Quart sized Pyrex pot

Heat the oil until just below simmering or very hot. Add your herbs, (be especially careful with fresh herbs as their natural moisture will cause the oil to pop) and place in a low 170 degree oven for about 2 hours. Let cool and strain off into sterile bottles. An extra sprig of herb can be added for esthetic purposes, but the medicinal properties of the plant will have already been rendered in the oil.

Ointment Variation: To make an ointment which is solid at room temperature follow the same formulation directions as shown above, only add 1 oz of beeswax or jojoba wax after straining off the herbal material and before pouring into jars.

Standard dosage: Infused oils may be taken internally when being used in cooking and flavoring dishes. Oil infusions are wonderful as massage oils to which Aromatherapy essences may also be added. Ointments don't run all over and are easily used for massage and healing of minor skin irritations.

Note: A few drops of benzoin tincture or essential oil can be added to any of the products designed for external use. It acts as a natural preservative without adding chemicals. You may also wish to store your finished products in the refrigerator as they will keep for several months under these ideal conditions.

Poultices and Compresses

Swatch of cheesecloth or herbal tea bag

1/2 oz of herbs

Poultices and compresses are easily made and suitable for topical application. An easy compress or poultice can be made using an herbal tea bag of choice, steeping it and applying directly to the site. A compress can be made of a decoction or infusion applied warm to a cloth pad and then wrung out. Poultices can be made by filling a square of cheesecloth with steeped or boiled herbs and applying while warm. After the poultice has cooled, it must be discarded as re-heating will not restore its medicinal properties. Native American people made poultices out of ground cornmeal and herbs, heated together and molded warm into a pad. A pot of this herb and cornmeal mixture was set beside the patient and when one poultice cooled, another was immediately put on in its place.

Recommended use: Always test a poultice or warm compress first to make sure it is not too hot to avoid blistering the skin. Wrapping the herbs in cotton gauze or strips will help to prevent loose herb material from entering a wound or break in the skin.

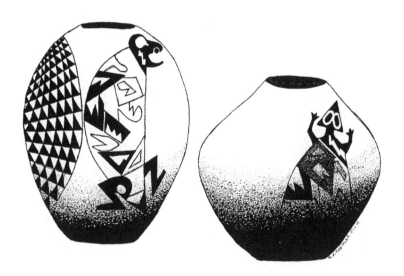

Herbal Recipes for: Skin, Hair and Body Care

Skin Care

"Yucca Root was used by Native tribes inhabiting the dry southwest desert regions to prevent body odor. Scarcity of water made bathing almost impossible."

Corn Meal Bath Scrub

1/2 cup blue cornmeal

1 tablespoon raw honey

1/2 cup Goldenseal tea, (tepid)

1 tablespoon of Cold Pressed Almond oil

Mix the cornmeal, honey and Goldenseal tea together and take the bowl into the bath with you. Get into the tub and take a moist handful of the scrub and begin massaging it all over your wet skin. Don't apply too much pressure, simply rub in soft circular motions paying special attention to your heels elbows and knees. Rinse with tepid water to remove all traces of the cornmeal. Now apply the cold pressed almond oil to your beautifully polished skin. Your body will feel newborn soft. Use this scrub at least once a week to keep your skin exfoliated and glowing

Note: A variation on this would include the use of an infused herbal oil such as marigold, rose or chamomile oil made with the same cold pressed almond oil.

Herbal Facial Cleanser

4 oz. of liquid unscented soap

1/4 cup of distilled water

1/4 cup of marigold infusion

1/4 cup of chamomile infusion

10 drops of essential oil of lavender

Mix all liquids together and store in an amber or cobalt blue bottle. The lavender and marigold are especially soothing and beneficial to the skin by speeding the regeneration of skin cells.

Variations-

*Rose Facial Cleanser-same formula as above, but add essential oil of rose instead of the lavender.

*Squash Facial Cleanser-In a blender, puree 1 small summer squash. Strain out any large bits of vegetable matter. This replaces the 1/4 cup distilled water in the Herbal Facial Cleanser formula. Keep refrigerated for up to a week.

*Corn Meal Facial Scrub-Simply add 1 teaspoon of blue cornmeal to any of the above formulas for a gentle, yet very effective exfoliating scrub.

Antiseptic Pine Acne Cleanser

4 oz. liquid, unscented Neutrogena soap

1/4 cup of pine needle infusion or10 drops of essential oil of pine in 1/4 cup of water

1 tbs. glycerin

Since all ingredients are liquid, mix and store in an amber bottle. Works well for acne pimples which tend to become infected. Also helpful in psoriasis conditions.

Variation: To make this into a natural antibacterial hand soap, add 5 drops of essential oil of eucalyptus to your unscented liquid soap.

Skin Healing Wash

4 oz liquid unscented Neutrogena soap

1/4 cup of chamomile infusion

1/4 cup of juniper infusion or 5 drops of essential oil of juniper

5 drops of essential oil of myrrh

The chamomile is soothing to the skin and the juniper, myrrh combination are healing for eczema and acne outbreaks. For severe cases, the wash can be left on for up to one minute and then thoroughly rinsed with tepid water.

Witchhazel Toner

1/8 cup of witchhazel

1/8 cup of lemon juice or 2-3 drops of lemon essential oil in 1/8 cup of water

1 cup of marigold infusion

Mix all strained infusions together and keep refrigerated

in a dark amber bottle. Sweep skin with a small amount on a cotton ball to remove all traces of makeup and cleanser residue. The lemon helps to restore the natural acid mantle the skin has to protect it from bacteria. The marigold balances out the formula by being very helpful for dry skin.

Note: Not for use on very dry or sensitive skin.

Gentle Mint Toner

1/4 cup of peppermint infusion

1 cup of marigold infusion

Make your infusions and strain. For best results keep in the refrigerator or in a cool place. Apply to a cotton ball or pad and sweep gently over face and neck after cleansing.

Most Gentle Rose Toner

1/2 cup of rose petal infusion or 5 drops of rose essential oil in 1/2 cup of water

1/2 cup of marigold infusion or 5 drops of marigold essential oil in 1/2 cup of water

1 tablespoon of liquid glycerin

Strain and combine your infusions and then add the tablespoon of glycerin as directed. This toner is very moisturizing and similar to the rose water and glycerin formulas of Victorian grandmother's time.

Natural Native Moisturizer

2 tablespoons glycerin

3 drops essential oil of rose

3 drops essential oil of marigold

1/4 cup comfrey infusion

Make your comfrey infusion or tea and mix it with the other ingredients. Shake well. Use as you would any other moisturizer.

Native Skin Nourisher

1 tablespoon of honey

1 tablespoon of glycerin

3 drops of essential oil of lavender

1/2 cup chamomile tea/infusion

After mixing all components together apply to freshly washed skin as a nighttime moisturizer and revitalizer.

Clover Blossom Bath Oil

1 cup of clover blossom oil infusion

5 drops of lavender essential oil

10 drops of yucca extract, (optional for a foaming bath oil)

Shake together and add a capful just before getting into the tub. Be careful when getting in and out as it can make the tub very slippery.

Calendula After Bath Oil

1 cup of marigold flower oil infusion

5 drops of ylang-ylang essential oil

5 drops of neroli or orange blossom essential oil

Shake oils together to combine for a skin soothing, uplifting treat after your bath or shower.

Note: Calendula is another name for marigold which is good for dry skin, healing of rashes and even varicose veins.

Natural Deodorant

1 cup coriander seed infusion

10 drops of essential oil of lemongrass

5 drops of essential oil of lavender

Place combined products in a glass spray bottle or atomizer. Unlike most anti-perspirants, it will not clog your pores. Spray under the arms and even the feet after a bath or shower.

Note: Yucca extract can be taken internally to inhibit odor causing bacteria. Native Americans in arid regions of the U.S. utilized this plant for just these purposes.

Natural Athlete's Foot Spray

1/4 cup juniper infusion or 5 drops of juniper essential oil in one pint of water

1/4 cup of Tea Tree infusion or 5 drops of Tea Tree oil in 1 pint of water

Amber glass spray bottle or atomizer and spray your feet lightly after bathing. Can be used to spray the floor of a public shower room before using to kill athlete's foot fungus.

Variation: You can add a few drops of both juniper and Tea Tree to any body or foot powder. Simply remove the sprinkle cap, add your essential oils to the powder and replace the cap. Shake to mix the oils thoroughly with the powder. Avoid cornstarch based powders whose naturally occurring sugars tend to only "feed" the fungus.

Natural Douche

1 pint of Cedarwood infusion, or 5 drops of essential oil of cedarwood (do not use if pregnant)

5 drops of Tea Tree oil

Combine products into a pint douche bag or applicator. The cedarwood is very helpful for most any vaginal infection and the Tea Tree oil is effective for candidiasis or yeast infections.

Note: A hot white willow bark douche has been traditionally used by Native American midwives for centuries to arrest bleeding after childbirth or post partum hemorrhage.

Natural Tooth Powder

1/4 cup Baking Soda

1/4 tsp. of ground myrrh or 5 drops of essential oil of myrrh

1/4 tsp. of finely ground peppermint leaves or 3 drops of essential oil of peppermint

Combine together and store in an airtight Tupperware container. Dip your wet toothbrush into the powder to use or sprinkle a little into the palm of your hand. Great for inhibiting the formation of plaque and freshening the breath.

Natural Mouthwash

1/2 cup of cooled peppermint infusion

1/2 cup of cooled basil infusion

2-3 drops of neroli or orange blossom essential oil

Mix the infusions together and add essential oil. Shake thoroughly, split the formula into two equal parts and keep one part refrigerated until use for best results. The basil and neroli are both wonderful for gum infections and mouth ulcers. The peppermint too gives you a pleasant lift in the morning!

Natural Native Hair Care

Soapweed Natural Shampoo

4 Tablespoons of dried, ground soapweed
(Yucca-root)

2 Tablespoons of dried mint leaves

1 piece of cheese cloth

Place herbs inside the cheese cloth and bring four
corners together. Tie a piece of string around the
opening and put in a mixing bowl. Pour 2 cups of
boiling water over the herbs and cover tightly. Let stand,
refrigerated, for 5 days, mixing gently each day. Pour over
hair to use and massage in. Rinse out with cold water.

Shine Enhancing Shampoo

4 Tablespoons dried soapwort
(sweet William)

2 Tablespoons dried rosemary

1 Cup of water

Place herbs in a sauce pan and cover with water.
Simmer for 5 minutes. Let stand until
cool. To use, massage into hair and scalp.
Rinse with cold water.

"The sweetness of Maple syrup is legend to have been discovered by an Indian maiden. Some of the tree's sap dripped into a hollow and mixed with freshly fallen rain. The young girl came by for a drink and found a unique sweetness mixed with the water. She told her people and they began tapping the trees and boiling the sap to make maple syrup.

Maple Deep Conditioning Treatment

2 Tablespoons pure maple syrup

2 Tablespoons lard

1/2 Teaspoon of honey

Place all ingredients into a small sauce pan and heat until melted and well incorporated. Let cool to a temperature that will be comfortable to apply to your scalp. Massage well, making sure to distribute throughout hair. Leave on 25 to 30 minutes. Shampoo out. note: if you have long hair, you may need to double this recipe.

Pumpkin Conditioner

1/2 Cup cooked pumpkin

1 Tablespoon lard

2 Tablespoons honey

1 Teaspoon dried rosemary

Starting with the pumpkin, place it into a clean blender or food processor. Blend until almost liquefied. Add additional ingredients and blend 5 minutes more or until well incorporated. Use as a mask on your hair, being sure to work it in well at the ends of your hair. Leave on for 20 to 25 minutes. Shampoo out and rinse well with cold water.

Hair Darkening Tonic

6 Tablespoons chopped rosemary

1 Tablespoon chopped sage

2 1/2 Cups boiling water

Turn heat off under water when it comes to a boil and place rosemary and sage in. Let steep over night. Be sure to strain this mixture before using it and to keep it refrigerated for no longer then five days. Use as a final rinse. Should not be used on light brown/blonde hair.

Fresh Mint Hair Rinse

1 Cup of fresh mint leaves

2 Cup of water

Lightly simmer for about 15 minutes. Turn heat off and let mixture stand until completely cool. Be sure to strain before using. Massage into scalp after shampooing and conditioning. Do not rinse out. Invigorating and stimulating for dry itchy scalp.

Hair Restoring Rinse

1/4 cup of Rosemary

1/4 cup of Nettle

1/4 cup of Cayenne Pepper or Capsicum

1/2 cup Sage

Steep for 10-15 minutes and let cool. This tonic may be used as a final rinse or applied to the scalp daily with a cotton ball. The cayenne is what encourages growth and when you stop using it, the rate of growth will again slow down. The other herbs help to nourish the scalp and give the hair a rich, brilliant shine.

Hair Strengthening Conditioner

1/2 box of plain Knox Gelatin

1/4 cup of chamomile

1/4 cup of ocean kelp or bladderwrack

Steep the chamomile and ocean kelp into an infusion for about 5-10 minutes and let cool. Next, prepare the gelatin as per the directions on the box and set aside. Combine the gelatin and herb mixture and apply as a final rinse or conditioner. Leave on the hair for about 3-5 minutes and rinse with cool water to close the cuticle of the hair. The gelatin helps strengthen the hair and reduce breakage and the kelp-chamomile blend adds revitalizing minerals.

Note: Individuals with a hypoactive (underactive) thyroid, often exhibit thin, dry hair which breaks easily.

Kelp has long been recommended as natural way to supply organic iodine, an essential nutrient necessary for normal thyroid function.

Hot Oil Treatment for Dry, Breaking Hair

1 tbs. of castor oil

10 drops of essential oil of bergamot

1 tbs. of sweet almond oil

Mix your oils in a little cup. Place your cup inside of a larger container which is filled with very warm water. Let the oil heat up and smooth onto the hair from roots to ends. Pin hair on top of the head and cover with a plastic bag for 15-20 minutes. For extra deep penetration cover the bag with a hot towel. Rinse, shampoo and use conditioner as usual. Castor oil is known to strengthen the hair shaft and prevent further breakage. The bergamot adds shine and elasticity by removing past product residues from the hair.

Mineral Hair Masque

1/4 cup bentonite clay

1/4 cup rosemary infusion

1/2 cup of sage infusion

Make a paste of the herbal infusions and dry bentonite clay which is available at many health food stores. Add or leave out a little extra water to make the hair masque to the desired consistency. Apply to hair with a spatula, top with a plastic bag and cover with a warm towel.

Rinse thoroughly after 15-20 minutes. Follow with a cool water rinse. The minerals from both the herbs and the clay will absorb into your hair, strengthening it and adding shine.

Light Hair Pomade

1/4 cup sweet almond oil

5 drops of oil of bergamot

1 oz beeswax

Melt all of the oils and beeswax together until liquefied. Add essential oil of bergamot and fill into sterile jars. No need to strain! Cap, cool and enjoy.

Variations: To add luster to dark hair add 1/4 cup of infused sage oil. To add highlights to light hair add 1/4 cup of infused chamomile oil.

Special Time Honored Remedies

here are secret formulas of Native American herbology so old, that we can not remember who first discovered it! Nonetheless they have stood the test of time for safety and effectiveness. This is an old formula similar to one that my mother used on my hair as a child to darken it and add shine. Much more than cosmetics, this salve is effective on everything from diaper rash to skin irritations and even scalp disorders. Here's how to make:

Little Crow's Soothing Salve

4 oz beeswax

2 ounces sesame oil

2 ounces almond oil

1/2 cup dried Indian Hemp (Brazilian Jaborandi)

1/2 cup dried Golden Seal Root (Hydrastis canadeis)

1/2 cup dried Sage Leaves (Saliva officinalis)

1/2 cup dried Red Clover blossoms (Trifolium prantense)

1/2 ounce liquid vitamin E

Using a glass pyrex pot, gently heat the beeswax and oil together until liquefied. Now carefully add your dried, ground herbs to the warm oil. Carefully remove from the stove, cover and place in a low oven, about 170 degrees F. for about four hours. When the time is up, remove from the oven and strain using a wire mesh sieve to remove herbal plant material. Add vitamin E, pour into jars, let cool until solidified, cap and enjoy!

This is a basic formula for any salve products, so just keep the proportions of 2 cups of dried herbs to 4 1/2 ounces of oil total.

Plantain Leaf Salve

3 Cups of fresh plantain leaves, finely chopped

4 oz. of olive oil

1/2 oz vitamin E

2-4 oz beeswax

The quintessential weed indeed! The common plantain was called "white man's foot" by many tribes because it seems to spring up where ever the settlers walked. Although not native to Native America, plantain was adopted as a useful herb for American Indians. Another good all purpose salve, plantain is especially good for diaper rash, itchy bug bites, and other skin irritations. For minor wounds it checks bleeding, speeds healing and takes the pain out of the scrape. Traditionally, raw leaves were ground into a soothing herbal poultice for use on burns.

Comfrey Salve

2 Cups of comfrey root

4 oz. of olive oil

1/2 oz vitamin E oil

2-4 oz. beeswax

5-10 drops benzoin

Prepare as other salves but chop or grind the comfrey roots well for maximum extraction of medicinal properties. Comfrey root has a high concentration of allantoin which causes a quick turnover and regeneration of skin cells. It is acclaimed for strengthening the skin tissues, making them more resilient and less prone to abrasions and tears. It is indispensable as a wound healer with unparalleled success in treating a myriad of skin complaints.

Red Clover Salve

2 Cups of red clover leaves and blossoms

4 oz. of olive oil

1/2 oz vitamin E

2-4 oz. beeswax

5-10 drops benzoin

Prepare as for a regular salve. Red clover has been investigated as being useful for cancer patients. Even more the leaves contain phytoestrogens which help to balance delicate female hormones benefiting the reproductive organs as well. The vitamin and mineral rich salve can be applied to the body after a bath or shower to stabilize hormone production in a similar way women use wild Mexican yam or progest creme.

Recipes for the Home:

Native American peoples have a special fondness for fragrant herbs used to scent the home. Smudges of sage are employed especially today for air purification and fragrancing.

Herbal smudges are done by burning the dried herbs of choice. Similar to incense, the smoke carries the chemical properties of the plant into the air. They are traditionally used in sweat lodge therapy, cleansing of air before a birth, celebration of marriage and many other important events. These formulas use all natural, organic materials and will not leave behind unwanted chemicals or propellants as do aerosol room fresheners. The naturally occurring botanical oils will kill airborne germs and leave a calming odor in your environment.

Pine Room Freshener

10 pine cones

Enough water to cover pine cones

Place pine cones in a large pot and fill with cold water until just covered. Let stand in water over night. Bring to a boil for 30 minutes. You can either leave on the stove above very low heat to disperse the scent or place cooled solution into a spray bottle. If using the first method make sure to never leave it unattended or on when out of the house. Also keep out of the reach of children.

Aromatic Pine Blend

2 Cups of broken up pine cones

1 Cup pine needles chopped

1/2 Cup rosewood chips (optional)

10 drops of cedarwood essential oil

Place broken pine cones and rosewood chips into a thick plastic bag. Pound with a hammer until well incorporated. Add pine needles and essential oils and mix well inside of bag. You can use the mixture in one of three ways. 1.) Take small cloth bags and fill with mixture. Tie off top and make a small loop. Hang anywhere that you want to be pleasantly scented. 2.) Put a large pot filled with water on the stove. Turn heat to low and let water come to a simmer. Add half of the blend and let steep in pot. The steam will carry the smell of the Pine Blend throughout your house. Remember to never leave the stove unattended or on when your out of the house. 3.) Take a large pottery or ceramic bowl and place mixture inside. The bowl can be left on your coffee table or anywhere that needs freshening. When you notice scent starting to dissipate, give the blend a few stirs with a spoon and add a few drops of cedarwood essential oil.

Cedarwood Pouch Blend

2 Cups cedarwood chips

1/2 Cup dried rosemary

1 Cup rosewood chips

5 drops cedarwood essential oil

Break wood chips up into small pieces. Add rosemary and essential oil of cedarwood. Using small cloth squares, place a mound of mixture in the center. Bring the four corners together and tie off with a piece of string leaving a small loop. Hang up in your closet to help repel moths or anywhere for a nice scent. Pouches can be made any size and re-scented with a few drops of cedarwood essential oil.

Pine Needle Fire Place Sticks

1 Cup chopped pine needles

1/2 Cup powdered rosewood

1 teaspoon benzoin gum

5 drops pine essential oil

enough water to make a paste

Grind pine needles in a blender until finely chopped. In a bowl mix together powered wood, essential oil, gum and water to form a thick paste. Using thick brown paper, place paste inside, spread out and roll paper tightly to form a thin stick. Moisten edge of paper with water and smooth so that the seam is sealed. Let sticks cure in a cool, dry place for 1 week. Once completely dry, use in your fireplace for a great aromatic treat. The size of paper that is used will determine the number of sticks able to be produced.

Cattail Aromatic Pillow

10 x 8 rectangle piece of clothe, preferably cotton

1 Cup broken up dried cattails

5 to 10 drops cedarwood essential oil

Mix cattails and cedarwood oil together. Let sit in a zip-lock bag for up to a week to allow the oil to permeate the cattails. Take cloth and fold over right sides together. Sew up 2 sides and turn pillow inside out. Fill pillow with cattail mixture and sew up the remaining open side. If you would like to be able to reopen your pillow to re-scent it, you can sew buttons across the top and close it that way. Larger pillows can be made to what ever size and shape you like.

Sweet Grass Blocks

1/2 Cup dried sweet grass shredded

1/2 teaspoon benzoin gum

3 Tablespoons powdered orris root

1 teaspoon powdered sugar

enough water to form a thick dough

1 charcoal disk

In a mixing bowl combine all ingredients well. Add

water to make a thick dough that can be molded by hand into little 1 inch blocks. Place onto a cookie sheet and set outside in the sun to dry. It can also be placed in a low oven until dry. Once dry to the touch store in a tin container for one week to cure. To use, heat charcoal which is made for incense over a burner of your stove. Use metal tongs and do so until the charcoal is ashed over. Place on ceramic plate or inside an incense burner. Use one Sweet Grass block at a time. The charcoal keeps the block burning and releasing its scent.

Pine Needle Blocks

Fresh pine needles work best. Chop them up to release the essential oils inside. Prepare recipe as above substituting pine needles for sweet grass. Because pine needles don't mix as well as sweet grass you may find the need to add more orris root powder. Let cure as above before using.

Cedarwood Blocks

Use 1/4 cup powdered cedarwood in place of sweet grass. Instead of plain water use rose water for a sweet effect. Prepare recipe as above. You may find rolling balls easier than forming blocks with this variation. Let cure as above before using.

Naturally Dried and Scented Baskets

Small, natural, native style woven basket

Dye water color of choice

Essential oil of cedarwood or pine.

Botanicals must be boiled in a pot of water until water changes color. This can take 2 to 6 hours. Once cooled, strain off plant materials and add essential oil of choice. 15 to 20 drops will usually do nicely. Dip basket in for 15 minutes. Make sure basket is completely covered with dye. After 15 minutes remove and let dry on a metal rack in the sun or in a cool spot. This makes a wonderful gift that will keep it's scent and character for a long time.

Purple: Black Mulberry leaves and berries.

Brown: Walnut shells and sage.

Yellow: Goldenrod flowers and stems.

Orange: Dried onion skins.

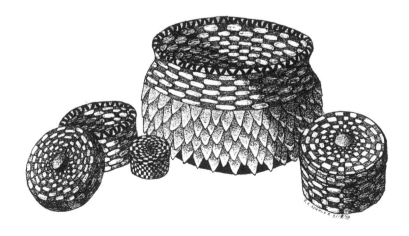

Scented Stones

2 Cups all purpose white flour

1 Cup water

1 Cup table salt

1 teaspoon white glue

2 to 4 drops of brown food coloring

In a large mixing bowl combine all ingredients and mix well with a wooden spoon. Sprinkle a little flour on a hard flat surface and turn dough out onto it. Knead a few times and divide into tablespoon sized amounts. Using your hands, roll and mold into stone shapes. Take a toothpick and draw a design on each stone. Place stones on a cookie sheet and bake at 300 degrees for about 1 hour. Remove and let cool on a cookie rack for 1 hour. In a large zip-lock bag add stones and essential oils of choice. Allow to cure for a week. Place in a ceramic or clay bowl for a great aromatic effect. When scent begins to dissipate, add more essential oil.

CHAPTER FOUR

FOOD IS MEDICINE
AND MEDICINE IS FOOD

Indigenous peoples do not distinguish between medicine and food as many are accustomed. Often times corn meal mush is given along with medicinal herbs as part of the total prescription for healing. To feed the body is to feed the soul! Many dishes can be classified as "comfort" foods because they bring us back to a place when we were healthy, happy and cared for. The emphasis here is to show that proper nutrition and enjoyment of food can and should go hand in hand, especially when illness strikes.

My mother and grandmother were exceptional cooks with my father being a most appreciative recipient! Native American men often encourage their wives cooking efforts and don't make a fuss when things don't turn out just right. Instead they praise the effort and give the cook confidence to try again, perhaps to do better next time. Wasting food was not to be done as well. Animals and plant life which provided sustenance were reverently appreciated as there are many thanksgiving ceremonies among the native American peoples and tribes. My father took pride in my mother's cooking saying she made the best roast turkey in town. To show his confidence, our home was often filled with visiting musicians, dignitaries, friends, family and neighbors, all served in our formal Victorian dining room. Our best china was never spared as my parents believed material things are destined to be used, not put in a showcase. I was taught to share and be genuinely gracious by offering guests refreshments and even a place to sleep if need be.

Food is just another extension of that hospitality as in tribal times the bounty of the hunt was divided appropriately by the entire camp, with no member going hungry. Therefore by feeding and healing ourselves, were are able to feed and heal our entire global community. In sharing this tradition you will see that once again these recipes give testament to the adaptability of American Indians to new foods by how we've incorporated them into our own style of delicious cuisine.

Corn Pancakes with Maple Syrup

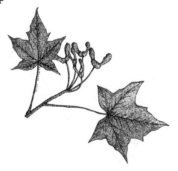

2 Cups milk

1 - 3 fresh eggs

1 teaspoon baking powder

1/2 teaspoon salt

2 Cups flour

3/4 Cup cooked corn

Mix all ingredients together except corn. Mix until only large lumps disappear. Add cooked corn. Pour onto lightly oiled medium to high skillet turning when small bubbles appear. Serve hot with butter and pure maple syrup which has been warmed. Yields about 16 - 4 inch pancakes. This was one of my favorites that my mother made me for cold winter mornings.

Variation:

Replace 3/4 cup cooked corn with 1 cup blueberries, blackberries or chopped apple.

Fried Cinnamon Apples

8 un-peeled cooking apples (Macintosh work well)

1/2 Tablespoon ground cinnamon

1/4 teaspoon nutmeg

1/4 Cup white sugar

1/4 Cup vegetable oil for frying

Cut your fresh apples into wedges, leaving the skins on. Cover with cinnamon, nutmeg and sugar. Set aside and cover. Begin heating your oil in a heavy skillet over medium - high flame. When a hint of smoke is present over the oil, it is time to add apples. Place in carefully. Cook until apples are golden and tender. Once done, let drain on a plate covered with paper towels. This was my paternal Aunt Laura's recipe from the Eastern Band Cherokee. When I slept over, this would be part of the morning fare.

Oh-No-Kwa (Hominy Grits)

Box of Hominy grits

maple syrup

butter or margarine

milk

Follow the directions given for preparation on box of grits. As grits begin to thicken, add your butter, maple syrup and milk to taste. Served this way, it makes a nutritious and tasty change from hot oatmeal. This is my brother Vance's favorite even today.

Variations:

Cornmeal can be substituted for the hominy grits.

Sapan (Lenape – White Cornmeal Gruel)

3 and 1/2 Cup milk

1 and 1/4 Cups white cornmeal

1 and 1/2 Cups maple syrup

butter

Boil the milk, stirring constantly over medium-high flame. Now add the white cornmeal and mix in the maple syrup. Lower the flame and keep stirring constantly to avoid lumps. A whisk will do well for this application. You can add butter and top with extra maple syrup, if desired. Serves 8 hearty appetites.

Anakee's Mulberry Muffins

1 Cup whole wheat flour

1/2 Cup quick oats

1/2 Cup brown sugar

1 Teaspoon baking powder

3/4 Cup fresh Mulberries

1/2 teaspoon salt

1 egg

1/4 Cup cooking oil

3/4 Cup milk

Preheat oven to 400 degrees. Combine all dry ingredients and form a well in the center. Mix egg, milk and oil together well and add to the well in the dry ingredients. The key is not to over mix. Leave it a bit lumpy. Add your fresh mulberries and pour into oiled muffin tin. Bake for 20 to 25 minutes. Yields: 1 dozen.

Variations:

Other fruits such as wild strawberries or blueberries can be used in place of mulberries.

Corn Bread (squares or muffins)

3/4 Cup yellow or white cornmeal

3/4 Cup whole wheat flour

3 teaspoons brown sugar or honey

1 tablespoon baking powder

1/2 teaspoon salt

1 egg

1/4 Cup cooking oil

3/4 Cup milk

Preheat oven to 425 degrees. Beat together egg, butter and milk. In another bowl combine dry ingredients. Quickly mix wet ingredients with dry, making sure not to mix too much. Try to leave it a bit lumpy. Fill your greased 8 x 8 pan for 16 squares or muffin tin and bake for 15 to 20 minutes. Delicious served with honey and butter.

Pumpkin Bread

1 and 3/4 Cup whole wheat flour or a mixture of 1 Cup whole wheat and 3/4 Cup all purpose.

1 teaspoon baking soda

1 teaspoon baking powder

1/2 teaspoon salt

1/2 teaspoon pumpkin pie spice / cinnamon / ginger

1/3 Cup milk

1 Cup cooked pumpkin

1/2 Cup oil or softened butter

2 eggs

1/2 Cup honey

Preheat oven to 350 degrees. Mix and prepare as other quick breads (mixing all wet ingredients together well, mixing dry ingredients separately, then adding the two together.) making sure pumpkin is well messed before adding to the wet mixture. Bake 1 hour for loaf or 25 minutes for muffins.

Grandmother "Hoosh's'" Light Rolls

Part 1:

1 Cup boiled milk

1/3 Cup sugar

1 Cup vegetable oil

Combine the above ingredients well... then mix with:

3/4 Cup ice water

1 beaten egg

Add 2 yeast packs (quick action) and next 1/4 cup lukewarm water. Combine the above with 3 cups of sifted flour. Let stand for about 20 minutes.

Part 2:

2 and 1/2 Cups flour

1 Tablespoon baking powder

1 and 1/2 teaspoon salt

1/2 teaspoon baking soda

Sift these all together and mix with part 1. Let stand in a warm place for one hour or until doubled in mass. Grease pans lightly and set oven to 350 degrees. Rolls can be shaped by lightly putting three balls in one muffin tin or rolling them into crescent shapes. Bake until they have fully risen and have a golden brown color, which can take about 20 minutes.

Cherokee Fry Bread

2 Cups self rising flour

1 and 1/2 Cups whole milk

Powdered sugar or honey

Pinch salt

Vegetable oil for deep frying

Sift your flour and add a pinch of salt. Slowly pour in milk. Work it into a ball and knead it until smooth and silky. Sprinkle a little flour on your table and roll it out. Cut 5 inch diameter circles and put a hole in the center. Place carefully into hot oil and let get golden brown and puffy. Serve with fruit preserves, powdered sugar or honey.

Variations:

Fresh blueberries can be added to the fry bread dough. 1/4 to 1/2 cup.

Broiled Tomatoes

3 pounds ripe tomatoes

1 medium green pepper

2 slices of bread (for crumb topping)

1 Tablespoon butter

1/4 Cup sugar

Cut and quarter tomatoes. Dice the green pepper finely and add the sugar. Set aside. Break the bread into crumbs. Put tomatoes and peppers into a sauce pan and cook adding 1/4 cup of water for about 10 minutes. Turn tomatoes out onto a oiled broiling pan and place in a broiler for about 15 minutes, topping with crumbled bread crumbs. Cook at 500 degrees or broiler setting.

Baked Sweet Potatoes

6 Medium sweet potatoes (long, skinny ones tend to be sweeter)

honey

corn oil or butter

Wrap the oiled potatoes in aluminum foil and bake in a 400 degree oven for 1 hours. Cut open foil, add butter and honey and re-wrap until ready to serve. Sweet potatoes have hormone balancing properties for menopausal women and should be included in the diet, perhaps more than white potatoes. An added bonus is the high amount of the super antioxidant vitamin, beta-carotene.

Baked Pumpkin

1 small pumpkin

2 Tablespoons maple syrup

1 teaspoon pumpkin pie spice

2 Tablespoons apple cider

1 Tablespoon butter

cinnamon

Preheat oven to 350 degrees. Cut a small pumpkin in half and place in the oven for 1 and 1/2 hours. When done, scoop out the pumpkin meat from shell and mash adding maple syrup, spice, apple cider and butter. Return filling to pumpkin shell, topping it with a little cinnamon and bake another 30 minutes. Don't throw away the seeds. My cousin Debbie use to toast the seeds after boiling them in a little salted water. She would spread them flat on a tray after boiling and toasting them for about 30 minutes at 350 degrees.

Aunt Lizzy's Potatoes

6 - 7 frying potatoes

1 medium green pepper

1/4 Cup cooking oil

1 onion

1 clove minced garlic (optional)

salt and pepper

Slice potatoes into rounds, like potato chips only a little thicker. Heat the cooking oil in the skillet on a medium-high flame. Add the potatoes and after they begin to brown, add the sliced onion and green pepper. The garlic should be added next, prior to serving because it tends to burn easily. When done, blot on paper towels and add salt and pepper to taste. My Great Aunt Lizzy was my maternal grandfather's sister and lived to be over 100 years old!

Mom's Crookneck Squash

6 - 8 yellow Crookneck squash or Zucchini

1 medium onion

1/4 Cup cooking oil

salt and pepper

Slice the squash into about 1/2 inch rounds. Chop the onion. Preheat the frying pan with the oil and add the squash and the onion. Sauté for about 15 minutes or less. You want the skin of the squash to be tender. Add salt and pepper to taste. My favorite part of the dish was the cooked squash seeds.

Pow Wow Corn Soup

3 pounds cubed beef

1 Cup chopped tomatoes

1 Cup red kidney beans

1 Cup white hominy

1/2 inch thinly sliced fatback

1 Cup chopped green string beans

1 Cup corn

1 chopped onion

4 Cups water

Brown the cubed beef and onion in a little oil and put in a crock pot or Dutch oven with the rest of the ingredients. Cook until beef is tender (about 3-4 hours). Add salt and pepper to taste.

Birch Bark Chicken

1 chicken (cut up)

garlic powder

1 medium chopped onion

3/4 Cup water

1 can tomato paste

1 teaspoon sugar

1 teaspoon liquid smoke (optional)

Birch bark

Thin the tomato paste with 1/4 to 3/4 cup of water. Add garlic powder, chopped onion, sugar and liquid smoke to make the marinating sauce. Place chicken in sauce and coat well. Let sit in your refrigerator over night if possible. Start coals in your smoker or barbecue and when hot place birch bark on top. Mix the chicken around in sauce to coat well again and place on grill. Turn and cook until completely done.

Roast Corn

4 ears of fresh white sweet corn

4 Tablespoons butter

Aluminum foil

Shuck the corn and wrap ears in aluminum foil but before sealing, add 1 tablespoon of butter. Spread over length of corn. Seal tightly and lay on bare coals, turning continuously until done.

Skewered Scallops

1/2 Cup melted butter

1/2 Cup sunflower seed oil

2 dozen cherry tomatoes

3 minced garlic cloves

1 dozen small green peppers (halved)

1 dozen small onions

2 dozen Jerusalem Artichokes (scrubbed)

4 dozen sea scallops

Mix butter, oil and minced garlic together and set aside. Alternating scallops and vegetables on about 8 skewers, brushing them with oil mixture. Roast on the grill for 15 - 20 minutes or until scallops are opaque, basting them with the remaining oil. Serve with fresh parsley and dill weed as garnish.

Roast Cornish Game Hen w/ Cornbread-Oyster Stuffing

2 Cornish Game Hens or 4 dressed quails

5 Cups toasted cornbread crumbs

1/2 stick butter

1 teaspoon Bell's seasoning or dried sage

2 cloves minced garlic

2 Tablespoons giblet broth or more for moister stuffing

1 Cup of cooked or canned oysters (save liquid)

Remove giblets and simmer in about 3/4 cup water for

20 minutes. Put stuffing ingredients in a bowl and melt 1/2 stick of butter to add in with 2 tablespoons or more of giblet broth. Now add onion, garlic, Bell's seasoning or dried sage, and oysters and stuff your hens. Place them on a rack in a roasting pan in a preheated 350 degree oven for about 1 hour 45 minutes or until legs move easily at the joints. A delicious gravy can be made from the pan drippings, reserved oyster liquid and giblet stock by combining them in a sauce pan and adding a tablespoon of flour more or less to thicken. A delicious alternative to roasted turkey for those special get together with family and loved ones.

Pumpkin or Winter Squash Pie

9 inch pie shell

2 Cups cooked, mashed pumpkin or squash

1/4 to 1/3 cup honey

1 Cup light cream

1 teaspoon pumpkin pie spice

1 teaspoon cinnamon

1 teaspoon ginger

Blend all filling ingredients until very smooth and creamy. Pour into pie crust and bake 55 minutes to 1 hour at 400 degrees or until a knife inserted in the center comes out clean.

Snow Ice Cream

8 Cups clean snow or shaved ice

1 Cup light cream

1 teaspoon pure vanilla extract

1/2 Cup maple sugar or syrup

Quickly blend snow in a cold bowl and add sugar, cream and vanilla to serve immediately. My mom used to make this for us when the snow was quite a bit cleaner!

Maple Walnut Cookies

1/2 Cup melted butter

1/2 Cup brown sugar

1/2 Cup white sugar

1 teaspoon maple extract or syrup

1 teaspoon salt

1 and 1/2 cup whole grain or wheat flour

1 egg

1/2 teaspoon baking soda

1/4 Cup walnuts

Preheat oven to 335 degrees. Mix wet and dry ingredients separately, then pour the wet into the dry mixture. Drop by tablespoons onto a pre-oiled cookie sheet and bake for 12 minutes.

Refreshing Herbal Teas

erbal teas can be used therapeutically to help heal the body or used constitutionally for nutrition and enjoyment. Served hot or iced, they provide variety, flavor and a much better alternative to caffeinated beverages and fruit drinks. They can compliment a meal by helping to aid in digestion or provide a quiet prelude to the evening's winding down from a hectic day. Many of the blends will help assist hormonal balance, weight loss, restful sleep, mental alertness and increased energy without central nervous system stimulation.

All of these teas are steeped as standard infusions for 3–5 minutes or more to suit your taste. Remember, the longer you steep, the more bitter, yet beneficial plant tannins you will extract from the herb. Tannins are thought to be phytochemicals which allow a plant to protect itself from insects. It is the dark brown sediment in the bottom of your cup if you've steeped your tea for a long time. Some herbs are less palatable than others, so a little raw honey or maple syrup can even be added to improve the taste. Adding sweeter herbs such as chamomile, raspberry, huckleberry or other berries to your mix will greatly improve the flavor while adding medicinal value and nutrition. Remember never to re-boil water for making herbal teas or your end product will be flat tasting due to the depletion of the oxygen in the first boiling.

Native Woman's Blend

1/2 cup of dried red raspberry leaves and berries

1 tsp. powdered wild yam root

1/4 cup of dried red clover blossoms

1/4 cup of dried chamomile

Mix the dried herbs and powdered root together into a dry blend. To brew use a ball and steep 1 oz of blend in one pint of water for 2-5 minutes, (standard infusion). This blend is rich in hormone balancing phytoestrogens and bioflavanoids. It also contains rich amounts of easy to absorb calcium, magnesium, B-complex vitamins and minerals. Wonderful for PMS, menopause and beyond!

Natural Fertility Blend

1/2 cup of red raspberry leaves

1/2 cup of dried red clover blossoms

Shake the blend together and make a light infusion. Red clover is very nutritious and is thought to help balance the delicate vaginal pH needed for sperm survival. The raspberry leaves and berries are also great for balancing female hormones and acts synergistically in this blend.

Native Pregnancy Tea

1/2 cup of dried red raspberry leaves and berries

1/4 cup of dried nettles

1/4 cup dried red clover blossoms

This blend offers so much for the pregnant woman. The red raspberry is helpful for morning sickness and is reported to help prevent miscarriage. Nettles are rich in easy to absorb vitamins and minerals all properly balanced and bioavailable. Nettles also help with night leg cramps so common in pregnancy. The raspberry leaves contain fragrine, a uterine tonic which allows for a safe and comfortable childbirth experience.

Breastmilk Builder

1/4 cup red raspberry leaves

1/4 cup red clover blossoms

1/4 cup fennel seed

1/4 cup blessed thistle leaves

All of these herbs are highly nourishing galactogogues, (plants which increase milk flow) and will encourage the production of high quality breastmilk. Before the use of bovine hormones in dairies, farmers added fennel to their cows feed to naturally boost milk production.

Teepee Creepers Pleaser

1/4 cup of dried spearmint leaves

1/4 cup of dried red clover blossoms

1/4 cup of dried nettles

1/4 cup of dried elderberries

Mix all dried herbs together and store in a zip lock bag in the refrigerator. Can be served chilled or iced. Very pleasant tasting it offers vitamins, minerals and a healthy dose of vitamin C. Elderberry is now being investigated for its reported ability to thwart the common cold.

Midday Energizer

1/2 cup of dried peppermint leaves

1/2 cup of dried red clover blossoms

Shake your blend thoroughly to mix the clover and mint. The peppermint is mildly stimulating and will wake up both your brain and body. The red clover is rich in b-complex vitamins, nature's natural energy boosters. Try it instead of the usual afternoon cup of coffee or candy bar.

Cold Chaser Blend

1/8 cup of dried pine needles

1/2 cup of dried rose hips

1/8 cup of dried echinacea root

Blend all three dried herbs and drink hot at the first onset of a cold. The pine needles will relieve nasal congestion or the sniffles which often signal the start of a cold. The echinacea or purple coneflower boosts your immunity naturally by increasing white blood cells and their activity.

Note: Once a cold has set in, add 1/8 cup of dried goldenseal root to this blend to fight it.

To cool a fever, add 1/8 cup of spearmint or peppermint leaves to this blend.

Iron Tonic

1/4 cup of dried yellow dock root

1/4 cup of dried rose hips

1/4 cup of dried dandelion root

1/4 cup of dried alfalfa

The yellow dock and dandelion are very bitter so you can use a food processor or coffee mill to grind the herbs into a powder and then fill two piece gelatin capsules. This herb blend can be also made into a tincture and taken with orange juice. (See tincture instructions)

Note: The presence of vitamin C is needed for proper iron absorption, hence the addition of rose hips in this blend.

Tummy Soother

1/2 cup of dried chamomile

1/4 cup of dried catnip

1/4 cup of dried spearmint leaves

Mix your herbs together. Can be served with a meal to

help with digestion and may help to prevent stomach upset.

Ex-Gas Variation: For indigestion coupled with gas, add 1/8 cup of fennel seed to this blend.

Note: In India after a meal, fennel seed mixed with tiny candies is served. Collectively called "sweets", these make the perfect after dinner mint for their sometimes spicy cuisine.

Natural Calm Tea Blend

1/4 cup of dried alfalfa

1/4 cup of dried chamomile

1/4 cup of dried valerian root

1/4 cup of dried scullcap

This tea blend nourishes as it calms by providing calcium, magnesium and B-vitamins so important to central nervous system function. Use before bedtime as a hot beverage.

Note: To heighten relaxation, put a drop of pure essential oil of lavender on your pillowcase. You'll sleep like a baby!

Sunrise Herb Tea Blend

1/4 cup of dried marigold flowers

1/4 cup of dried elderberries

1/2 cup of dried rose hips

Full of vitamin C and brain waking phosphorus, this blend is great for getting you started in the morning.

Slimming Tea Blend

1/2 cup of dried watercress

1/4 cup of dried kelp

1/4 cup of dried chamomile flowers

The watercress and kelp contain naturally occurring, organic iodine which is crucial to the proper function of the thyroid. A sluggish or hypoactive thyroid can mean extra pounds of extra weight, dry skin and hair as well as an extreme sensitivity to coldness. An added bonus, this formula has a mild diuretic action, helping to quell excess water weight gain.

Natural Brain Power Blend

1/2 cup of dried basil

1/8 cup of dried rosemary

1/4 cup of dried peppermint leaves

This blend is based on an herb tea that my paternal aunt Laura would send me off with in the morning with one of her fabulous breakfasts. The peppermint wakes you up and stimulates digestion while the basil and rosemary heighten mental function and alertness. Wonderful as an aid for memory retention. It is truly brain food!

Note: Do not use at night unless you're cramming for an exam!

Blues Chaser Blend

1/2 cup blessed thistle leaves

1/4 cup St. John's Wort

1/4 cup red clover blossoms

This blend is excellent for depression caused by PMS, menopause, stress, etc. New research is pointing to imbalances in serotonin as the root cause of depression in women suffering from premenstrual syndrome and menopausal symptoms.

Note: Do not use St. John's Wort if you are on a SSRI or selective serotonin re-uptake inhibitor such as Zoloft, Paxil and Prozac. Used in combination with these medications, it can cause excessively high levels of this neurotransmitter in the body and increasing the drug's potential side effects such as sensitivity to sunlight.

Keep in mind that any and all of these blends can be rendered as herbal tinctures. Simply follow the instructions for making tinctures using the herbs and ingredients from each blend. Once made into a tincture, a quick, hot cup of herbal tea can be made very easily by adding 10-15 drops to a cup of water. If you are concerned about the alcohol content in a tincture, remember that the grain spirits act as a preservative and will evaporate off in the hot steam if you allow it to stand for a few minutes before drinking. Honey can be added to your herb teas to improve the flavor of more acrid blends but never give honey to very small infants as cases of botulism have been associated with its use in children under one year of age. Instead, you might try maple syrup as a safe and natural sweetening agent for younger ones.

Native American Kitchen Remedies

ver the centuries as native American peoples have become dispossessed from the land we have had to adapt to the resources available to us. As more and more people crowd into the cities, much is lost in respect to living off of the land. All the same newer products have been incorporated into kitchen remedies, some mixed with traditional herbs and others not.

The following home cures are from my paternal aunt Alberta of the Six Nations Iroquois. She spent much time close to my grandmother "Hoosh" learning much about how to heal and care for themselves with simple, inexpensive yet eminently effective kitchen treatments.

Onions for Colds and Fever

My aunt Alberta has used sliced raw onions placed inside of wool or cotton socks to break a fever and speed a cold on its way. Slice a fresh raw onion through the rings and place the onions inside of the socks positioned on the soles of the feet. She even recommends placing sliced onions in a dish in the room where the patient is staying. It is believed that the onions draw out the fever from head to toe. Allicin, one of the active components in both onion and garlic has been shown to inhibit the growth of microorganisms. Treatments placed on the soles of the feet are readily absorbed by diffusion through the skin, hence their time respected application.

Octagon Soap for Skin Irritations and Poison Ivy

Octagon soap has been an old standby for both personal and household cleaning for a number of years. Rustic and basic, this soap has a no-nonsense approach to getting the job done! My aunt suggests that nothing works better on itching skin due to contact dermatitis including poison ivy, oak and sumac reactions. A lather of the soap can be left on the skin to dry up such irritations quickly. Rinse off at the end of the day.

Aesthetic Badge to Ward Off Disease

An aesthetic badge was a swatch of cloth like cotton or muslin which was infused with paraffin, camphor, menthol and other herbs. During the smallpox epidemic of the 1800's many people sought to arm themselves with such herbal protections. In the 18th and early 19th century, many children wore a piece of camphor suspended from a string around their neck next to the skin. The aesthetic badge harkens from this same practice. The camphor, ground peppermint leaves and paraffin were melted together until liquid. Next it was poured warm onto the cotton cloth where it was absorbed. After the paraffin hardened, the cloth was cut into swatches and pinned on the inside of a child's undershirt. My cousin Carol, (aunt Alberta's daughter), remembers not wanting to wear it to school due to its "distinctive" odor but relinquished to wear it to bed! She said that she was never sick in any event and credits the badge for at least some part in that.

GLOSSARY

Acne: An inflammatory disease of the sebaceous or oil glands characterized by the eruption of pimples.

Alkaloids: medically noted plant compounds exhibiting nitrogen molecules in ring structures.

Analgesic: A product or compound which relieves pain.

Antibiotic: Substance that represses the growth of or kills micro-organisms.

Anti-fungal: Substance that destroys fungi.

Anti-inflammatory: Reduces or lessens swelling and inflammation.

Anti-oxidant: Slows or stops oxidation of tissues and substances.

Antipyretic: Helps to reduce a fever

Antiseptic: Helps to kill germs and bacteria.

Aromatic: A compound with a distinct aroma or tastes.

Astringent: A product which draws tissues together.

Bactericidal: Working to kill bacteria.

Berry: A small fruit with one main pit or many seeds. May contain poison.

Cleanser: A purifying wash.

Decoction: Product which is boiled to extract medicinal properties.

Detoxification: Neutralizing toxins or poisons.

Diuretic: Aiding in the excretion of excess bodily fluid.

Emetic: Induces vomiting.

Essential oil: A complex volatile oil which has been extracted from plants, seeds, flowers or roots.

Estrogen: A hormone associated with the female reproductive cycle produced in the ovaries.

Exfoliant: A compound which will remove the upper layer of dead skin cells.

Expectorant: Helps to loosen and expel phlegm and other material from the respiratory tract.

Germicidal: Active against germs.

Humectant: Brings moisture to the skin.

Hypotensive: Lowers blood pressure.

Infusion: Used when plant material is soft and easily extractable such as leaves and flowers. Hot water is used to steep.

Lipids: Fat-like substances such as waxes, fats and phospholipids.

Medicine Man: Native American traditional healers with a working knowledge of herbs.

Medicine Woman: Native American traditional healers which often include midwives.

Medicine Society: Secret healing society of the Iroquois Confederacy.

Mucous Membrane: The membranes which are moist and line the mouth, nasal passages, lungs, etc.

Nervine: Refers to the nervous system and how a certain substance may have a calming or stimulating effect.

Nutritive: Provides nutritional support.

Paturation: Childbirth.

Pharmacognosy: The study of medicines derived from plants and natural sources.

Pod: Dried plant matter usually in the form of a cylinder which splits open when ripe to disperse seeds.

Progesterone: Female hormone produced in the ovaries after the egg is released.

Relaxant: Induces calm and relaxation.

Sedative: Induces sedation or sleep by calming over-excitement of the nervous system.

Shaman: Medicine man of the Tibetan regions of Asia.

Smudge: Burning an herb and using the ashes for purification and disinfection.

Stimulant: Increases energy by exciting the central nervous system.

Steep: To allow an herbal product to brew for a period of time.

Tannins: Bitter phenolic-rich products found in the galls, leaves and barks thought to aid in the repulsion of insects.

Tonic: A medicine which increases strength and tone.

NATIVE HERB QUICK REFERENCE

Alder (*Alumus crispa*) Native peoples used this tree's bark for red dye. An acrid tea was also made that was traditionally used for stomach aches and colds.

Alum Root (Herchera americana) It's roots are astringent in their raw from. Tea from the roots was used to stop diarrhea.

Arbor Vitae (*Thuja occidentailis*) The natural volatile oils of this plant are an effective insect repellent.

Bay (*Laurus nobilis*) The leaves of the plant are well known for flavoring stews, but did you know that a few leaves placed in your favorite canister helps repel grain months?

Bee Balm (*Monarde didyma*) My aunt Laura's favorite. This fragrant herb of the mint family and must be boiled to extract flavor and qualities.

Black/Blue Cohosh (*Cimicifuga recemosa*) Roots make an excellent tea for use during childbirth. I've used it myself for that purpose and found it to be quite helpful.

Boneset (*Eupatorium perfoliatum*) More commonly used, is Indian sage. My people have used a strong tea from this herb to keep their black hair dark and lustrous as well as a stimulant for hair growth.

Cherry Bark (*Prunus virginiana*) The bark of this common tree contains hydrocyanic (prussic) acid and was and still is used as a cough suppressant.

Cattail (*Typha latifolia*) The roots or tubers of this free range plant and young shoots are edible. The "down" from inside the tail was used by settlers to stuff futons and pillows.

Cranesbill (*Geranium maculatum*) More commonly known as wild alum, the root was first dried to preserve it's astringent properties.

Damiana (*Turnera aphrodisiaca*) This tiny shrub has a strong aromatic quality. The leaves were used medicinally as a stimulant.

Dock (*Rumex hymenoseplus*) Often called wild spinach, these hardy perennial weeds grow profusely throughout the U.S. Cooked and eaten like spinach.

Dogbane (*Apocynum* and *rosaemifolim*) Found throughout the U.S. and Canada, the juice of this plants large milky roots were said to remove warts.

Elm (*Ulmus fulav*) Otherwise known as red or slippery elm. A tea made from the inner bark is an effective sore throat gargle.

Echinacea (*Brauneria angustifolia*) Used as a blood purifier and to counter the poison from snake and insect bites.

Fennel (*Foeniculum officinale*) Although a popular culinary herb, did you know that the tea made from the tea seeds helps dispel gas and comfort colic in babies?

Fringe Tree (*Chionanthus virginicus*) The outer root covering of this tree was used as a laxative and intestinal tonic.

Goldenseal (*Hydrastis canadensis*) The young shoots, fresh leaves and dried roots of this vine were used as a tea for kidney and urinary ailments.

Indian Tobacco (*Lobelia inflata*) The dried leaves were used medicinally and ceremonially by Native Americans but this is a potent narcotic plant that is highly poisonous.

Juniper (*Juniper virginiana*) Often called the eastern red cedar, the berries were boiled as a remedy for gout, dropsy and to hasten labor. Juniper berries have also been found to be an effective fungicide.

Linden (*Tilia americana*) Natives used the fibrous bark to make rope. The flowers and leaves make a fragrant tea for colds.

Live Oak (*Querous virginiana*) The acorns, which are highly toxic if eaten raw, contain tannic acid. The Native Americans removed it by a process and then the ground acorn meal was used as a nutritious base for venison stew.

Maple (*Acer sp.*) Native peoples were harvesting and processing maple sap into sugar long before the colonists arrived. It takes approximately 40 gallons of sap to produce 1 gallon of maple syrup.

Monard (*Monarde fistulosa*) A member of the mint family, it's leaves were incorporated into salves as a remedy for chest colds and congestion.

New Jersey Tea (*Ceanothus americanus*) Also called Indian tea, this native plant played a part in American history as the leaves were used as a substitute for English tea during the American revolution.

Pennyroyal (*Hedeoma pulegiodes*) My people used this plant's leaves as a tea for indigestion but it should never be used by pregnant women. When made into a salve, it's an effective insect repellent.

Poison Ivy (*Rhus redicans*) Yes, this was one of my many little surprises my people had waiting for the settlers. Strangely enough, I've never once heard of anyone in my family or myself contracting a rash from it even though it grows profusely in my hometown. The Native Americans method of immunity was to craw one of the tiny new leaves early in spring.

Raspberry (*Rhus ideaeus*) I can remember drinking this pleasantly ambrosial tea before the birth of my children. A tea of these leaves taken weeks before labor helps to increase the effectiveness of contractions.

Sassafras (*Sassafras officinale*) Twigs of this tree were used as an early toothbrush. The outer root covering was used as a spring tonic. The bark itself was good as an insect repellent.

Skullcap (*Scutellaria lateriflora*) The entire plant can be used to help calm frayed nerves and induce sleep.

Spikenard (*Aralia recemosa*) Similar in flavor to Queen Anne's Lace roots, the roots of this plant are used to flavor root beer. Natives used the roots as food and medicinally as cough medicine.

Trillium (*Trillium pendulum*) This plants roots were used therapeutically and has even found it's way into modern cancer research. It was once touted as an Indian love charm.

Turtlehead (*Chelone glabra*) This plant has pink-lavender flowers and was prepared as a tea for use as a vermifuge.

Witch Hazel (*Hammamel virginiana*) The inner bark was prepared as an infusion and a lotion was made from it which was very beneficial for skin problems.

Wintergreen (*Gaultheria procumbens*) Used primarily today as a mint flavoring, this herb contains salicylates which hold a similarity in formation to acetylsalicylic acid commonly known as aspirin. Native people used this plant for much the same purpose, to relieve pain and reduce fever.

Yerba Santa (*Eriodictyon californicum*) Literally translated as "Holy Herb" Native Americans taught the southwestern Spanish settlers how to use this beneficial plant. A tea was made for colds and respiratory complaints. The leaves were taken along and chewed during trips across the arid plains as a natural thirst quencher.

Conversion Chart

Dry:

    1/4 Cup – 4 Tablespoons – 2 ounces
    1/2 Cup – 8 Tablespoons – 4 ounces
    1 Cup – 16 Tablespoons – 1/2 pound – 8 ounces

Wet:

    1/4 Cup – 2 fl ounces
    1 Cup – 7 fl ounces
    25 drops essential oil – 1/4 teaspoon
    50 drops essential oil – 1/2 teaspoon

References & Resources

Helpful Books

The Scientific Validation of Herbal Medicine by Daniel B. Mowrey, Ph.D. Keats Publishing

An Introduction to Common Medicines 5th Edition by Dr. Glen Hanson, Department of Pharmacology & Toxicology, College of Pharmacy, University of Utah, Salt Lake City Utah 84112

The Healing Herbs by Micheal Castleman, Rodale Press

Internet

For more information on natural medicines, vitamins, herbs and pharmaceuticals, visit *The Interaction Profile* website at: **www.interactions.homepad.com.**

To Join Dr. Miczak's Native Community which features herbal medicine, forums and a lecture calendar, visit her *Native Traditions*' website at: **www.clubhomepage.com/native**.

Also, be sure to visit Dr. Miczak's Apothecary website at: **http://click-on.to/apothecary**.

Herbal Supplies

Herb Products Company

11012 Magnolia Blvd., P.O. Box 898
North Hollywood, CA 91603-0808

Credit Card Orders: (888) 339 HERB (4372)

Customer Service: (800) 877-3104
(818) 761-0351 of Fax (818) 508-6567

Bulk herbs, extracts, essential oils, clear gelatin capsules, oils and
more. Practically everything you'll need to make the products in this
book... all in one place. For more supplies and information stop by
Dr. Miczak's Apothecary website at
http://click-on.to/apothecary and visit the book and
"Cyber-Store."

Internatural

33719 116th St.-NW
Twin Lakes, WI 53181 USA

800-634-4221 (toll free order line)
262-889-8581 (office phone)
262-889-8591 (fax)

e-mail: internatural@lotuspress.com
website: www.internatural.com

Retail mail order and internet reseller of essential oils, herbs, spices
supplements, herbal remedies, incense, books and other supplies.

Lotus Light Enterprises

PO Box 1008-NW
Silver Lake, WI 53170 USA

800-548-3824 (toll free order line)
262-889-8501
262-889-8591
e-mail: lotuslight@lotuspress.com

Wholesale distributor of essential oils, herbs, spices, supplements, herbal remedies, incense, books and other supplies. Must supply resale certificate number or practitioner license to obtain catalog of more than 10,000 items

Native American News Journals and Magazines

News from Indian Country
7831 N. Grandstone Ave.
Hayward, WI 54843-2052

Akwesasne Notes
Mohawk Nation via Rooseveltown, NY 13683-2052

The American Indian Review

3 The Homesteads, Hunsdon, Ware
Herfordshire SG12 8QJ, England, UK

Native American Clothing and Crafts

Authentic Native American Dance Regalia by JoAnn "Sews-A-Lot"

(409) 866-5600 or (860) 763-5963

All sizes ribbon shirts, ladies shawls, ladies dresses, custom orders welcome, catalog available.

Wilderness Crafts

3 Andrews Rd., Dept. IC, Bath, ME 04530
(207) 442-8447

Drums, sage, hairpipe beads, plus other Native American crafts and supplies.

INDEX

Abscesses, - Willow bark for 41

Acidity pH 64

Acne - wash for 62

Alder *see quick reference*

Alfalfa - iron tonic 104

Alkaloids *see glossary*

Almond oil - Corn Meal Bath Scrub 61 , Hot Oil Treatment for Dry, Breaking Hair 73, Light Hair Pomade 74, Little Crow's Soothing Salve 75

Alum root *see quick reference*

Anakee's Mulberry Muffins 89

Analgesic *see glossary*

Anemia - dock for 22, iron tonic 104

Anthemis nobilis, *see* chamomile 65

Antibacterial 64

Antibiotic *see glossary*

Antifungal *see glossary*

Antipyretic *see glossary*

Antiseptic *see glossary*

Antiseptic Pine Acne Cleanser 62

Antispasmodics - sage 39, blue cohosh *see quick reference*

Apples, fried cinnamon 87

Arbor Vitae *see quick reference*

Aromatic *see glossary*

Aromatic Pine Blend 79

Arthritis - willow bark for stiffness 41, rheumatism 41

Artichoke, Jerusalem 30

Asprin 34, 41

Astringent *see glossary*

Athlete's foot spray 66

Aunt Lizzy's Potatoes 94

Baked Sweet Potatoes 93

Baked Pumpkin 93

Baking soda - natural tooth powder 68

Ball, tea 54

Balm of Gillead 2

Basic herbal products 53

Basil - Natural Mouthwash 68

Bath scrub - corn meal 61

Bay *see quick reference*

Beans, red kidney 95

Bee balm *see quick reference*, 15, 49

Beech, Wooster 6

Beechnut 14

Beech tree 14

Beeswax - Light Hair Pomade 74, Little Crow's Soothing
    Salve 75

Bentonite 73

Benzoin - Pine Needle Fire Place Sticks 80, Sweet Grass
    Blocks 81

Benzoin gum 77, 80

Bergamot - Hot Oil Treatment for Dry, Breaking Hair 73,
    Light Hair Pomade 74

Berry *see glossary*

Birch *see* black birch 16

Black and Blue Cohosh *see quick reference*

Black Birch 16

Bladder 21

Bladderwrack *see* kelp

Bleeding - Plantain Leaf Salve 16

Blessed Thistle leaves - Breastmilk Builder 102

Blood building *see* iron tonic

Blue Cohosh *see quick reference*

Blues Chaser blend 106

Blue cornmeal - Corn Meal Bath Scrub 61

Bile, sage for 39

Boneset *see* comfrey, *see quick reference*

Brazilian Jaborandi - Little Crow's Soothing Salve 75

Breaking hair 72, 73

Breath freshening 68

Breastmilk builder 102

Broiled Tomatoes 92

Burns, plantain leaf poultice for 76

Calcium - Native Women's Blend 101

Calendula *see* Marigold

Calming - Natural Calm Tea 105

Cancer, red clover for 37

Capsicum - red pepper 72

Carminative - elderberry 25

Cattail - Cattail Aromatic Pillow 19, 81

Caulophyllum *see* also cohosh

Castor oil 73

Cattail *see quick reference*

Cedarwood - Natural Douche 67, Aromatic Pine Blend
    79, Cedarwood Pouch Blend 80

Cedarwood Pouch blend 80

Chamomile - Herbal Facial Cleanser 62, Skin Healing Wash 63, Native Skin Nourisher 65, Hair Strengthening Conditioner 72, Native Women's Blend 101

Cherokee Fry Bread 92

Cherry bark *see quick reference*

Cherry, wild 20

Childbirth 9, 10, 18, 102

Children - Teepee Creeper Pleaser 102

Circulation of blood 25, 40

Cleanser *see glossary*

Clover *see* red clover 37

Coffin, Dr. 6

Colds 103

Colic - Tummy Soother 104

Comfrey - Salve 76, Natural Native Moisturizer 65

Compresses 59

Cone flower *see* echinacea

Corn 21 - Corn Pancakes with Maple Syrup 86

Corn Bread 89

Corn meal - White Cornmeal Gruel 88, Herbal Facial Cleanser 62

Corn Pancakes with Maple Syrup 86

Corn silk 21

Coughs 103

Cranesbill *see quick reference*

Damiana *see quick reference*

Dandelion - Iron Tonic 104

Decoction - *see glossary*, how to make 56

Detoxification - dock for 22

Depression - Blues Chaser Tea 106

Diabetes - Jerusalem artichoke for 30, nettle for 35

Diarrhea - antidiarrheal 113

Digestion 104

Disinfectants 78

Diuretics *see glossary*

Dock *see quick reference* 49

Douche 67

Dysmenorrhea 38

Dyspepsia 104

Echinacea - angustifolia 23

Eczema 75

Elder, Elderberry 25

Elm *see quick reference*

Elixir - tinctures, how to make 57

Emetic *see glossary*

Eruptions 63

Essential oil *see glossary*

Estrogen - female hormones *see glossary*

Exfoliant - Corn Meal Bath Scrub 61

Exhaustion - Midday Energizer 103

Expectorants *see glossary* - wild cherry 20

Eyes, goldenseal for 26

Face - *see* Native American Skin Care section 69

Facial cleansers 62

False face illustration 42

False Solomon's Seal 27

Female bleeding *see also* postpartum hemorrhage - willow for 41

Fennel *see quick reference*

Fertility - Natural Fertility Blend 101

Fevers, willow bark for 41

Flatulence - Tummy Soother 104

Fried Cinnamon Apples 87

Fringe Tree *see quick reference*

Garden - Native medicine wheel garden 46, garden planning 51

Gargles - Natural Mouthwash 68

Garlic 97

Gas 104

Germicidal *see glossary*

Goldenseal - Corn Meal Bath Scrub 61, *see quick reference*

Grandmother "Hoosh's" Light Rolls 91

Gums, care of 68

Hemorrhages 41

Hair - Natural Native Hair Care 69

Headaches - mint for 33, willow for 41

Hands - dry, chapped 76

Healing herb 75

Heart - beebalm for heart problems 15

Heartburn 104

Honey - Corn Meal Bath Scrub 61, Native Skin Nourisher 65, Maple Deep Conditioning Treatment 70, Pumpkin Conditioner 70

Humectant *see glossary*

Hydrangea 28

Hypotensive *see glossary*

Indian - sage *see quick reference*

Indigestion 104

Insomnia 105

Inulin 30

Iodine 73

Jerusalem Artichoke 30

Joints, stiff 41

Juniper - berries 29, Skin Healing Wash 63, *see quick reference*

Kelp - Hair Strengthening Conditioner 72

Kidneys see corn

Labor 39

Lactation 39, 102

Lactogogue also galactogogue 102

Lavender - Herbal Facial Cleanser 62, Native Skin
    Nourisher 65, Clover Blossom Bath Oil 65

Laxative 27

Lemon - Witchhazel Toner 63

Lemongrass 66

Linden *see quick reference*

Lipids *see glossary*

Live oak *see quick reference*

Lobelia inflata - Indian tobacco 3, 8

Lungs 27

Magnesium - Natural Calm Tea 105

Maize *see* corn

Maple 32, *see quick reference*

Maple syrup 86 - Maple Deep Conditioning Treatment 70

Marigold - Herbal Facial Cleanser 62, Witchhazel Toner
    63, Gentle Mint Toner 64, Most Gentle Rose Toner
    64, Natural Native Moisturizer 65, Calendula After
    Bath Oil 66

Medicine Man 3, *see glossary*

Medicine Woman 3, *see glossary*

Medicine Society 12, *see glossary*

Menopause symptoms 38

Menstruation - disorders, irregular, red raspberry for 38, Native Women's Blend 101

Miscarriage, prevention - Native Pregnancy Tea 102

Mint 49 - Natural Mouthwash 68, Fresh Mint Hair Rinse 71

Monard *see quick reference*

Mucous membrane *see glossary*

Mulberry Muffins 89

Muscular Aches 41

Myrrh - Skin Healing Wash 63, Natural Tooth Powder 68

Natural Athlete's Foot Spray 66

Natural Deodorant 66

Natural Douche 67

Natural Tooth Powder 68

Natural Mouthwash 68

Natural Native Hair Care 69

Nervice *see glossary*

Nettle 49 - Hair Restoring Rinse 11, Native Pregnancy

Tea 102, Teepee Creepers Pleaser 102

New Jersey Tea 49, *see quick reference*

Nutritive *see glossary*

Oh-No-Qwa - Hominy Grits 88

Oils - infused 58, olive, almond and sunflower 58

Orris root - Sweet Grass Blocks 81

Passionflower 50

Paturation *see glossary*

Pennyroyal *see quick reference*

Peppermint - Gentle Mint Toner 64, Natural Tooth
    Powder 68, Natural Mouthwash 68, Midday
    Energizer 103

pH 18

Pharmacognosy *see glossary*

Pine needles - Skin Healing Wash 63, Pine Room
    Freshener 78, Aromatic Pine Blend 79

Pine 78, 79, 80, 82

Psoriasis 63

Pine Room Freshener 78

Plantain 36

Plantain Leaf Salve 76

Premenstrual syndrome - blue cohosh for 17, Native Women's Blend 101, pumpkin, Pumpkin Conditioner 70, Pumpkin Bread 90

Pumpkin Bread 90

Pod *see glossary*

Poison Ivy *see quick reference*

Progesterone *see glossary*

Pure Food and Drug Act 6

Red Raspberry 38 - Native Women's Blend 101, Native Pregnancy Tea 102, Breastmilk Builder 102, *see quick reference*

Red Clover 37 - salve 75, Clover Blossom Bath Oil 65, Native Women's Blend 101, Natural Fertility Blend 101, Native Pregnancy Tea 102, Breastmilk Builder 102, Teepee Creepers Pleaser 102, Midday Energizer 103

Red Clover Blossom Bath 50, 65

Relaxant *see glossary*

Restlessness 105

Ringworm, dock for 22

Rose - Herbal Facial Cleanser 62, Most Gentle Rose Toner 64, Natural Native Moisturizer 65

Rosemary - Shine Enhancing Shampoo 69, Pumpkin

Conditioner 70, Hair Darkening Tonic 71, Fresh Mint
    Hair Rinse 71, Mineral Hair Masque 73, Cedarwood
    Pouch Blend 80

Rosewood chips - Aromatic Pine Blend 74, Cedarwood
    Pouch Blend 80, Pine Needle Fireplace Sticks 20

Sage 20 - Hair Darkening Tonic 71, Hair Restoring Rinse
    71, Mineral Hair Masque 73

Salves - making your own ointments 58, Little Crow's 75,
    Plantain 36, clover 37

Sapan - Corn Meal Gruel 88

Sassafras *see quick reference*

Scented stones 84

Sedative - wild cherry 20, goldenseal 26, red clover 37,
    skullcap 116, *see glossary*

Shaman 3, *see glossary*

Skin care *see* herbal recipes for skin

Skin irritations 58, 75

Skullcap *see quick reference*

Smudge *see glossary*

Soapweed *see* yucca

Soapwort 50 - Shine Enhancing Shampoo 69

Solomon's seal *see* false Solomon's seal

Spearmint 33

Spikenard *see quick reference*

Stomach - morning sickness 102,

Stones, aromatic 84

Stimulant *see glossary*

Steep *see glossary*

Sugar Maple *see* maple

Sunflower seeds 4

Sweet almond oil 73

Sweet grass blocks 81

Symphytum officinale *see* comfrey

Tallow, animal fat, lard 70

Tannic acid, tannins *see glossary*

Tea - refreshing herbal teas 100

Tea Tree - Natural Douche 67

Teeth - Natural Tooth Powder 68

Thyroid gland 73

Tonics *see glossary*

Toxins, purification of 25

Trifolium pratense *see* red clover

Trillium *see quick reference*

Tumors 37

Turtlehead *see quick reference*

Ulcerated sores 27

Urinary infections *see* corn silk for 21

Urine - diuretic 21

Urtica dioica *see* nettles

Uterine 38

Uterus 38

Vermifuge, beebalm 15

Vitamins 38

Vomiting, emetic *see glossary*

Weight reducing 106

White, willow *see* willow 41

Wild *see* cherry 20

Willow bark 41

Wounds *see* plantain 36, salve 76

Witch Hazel - Witchhazel Toner 63, *see quick reference*

Wintergreen *see quick reference*

Yerba Santa *see quick reference*

Yucca root - Clover Blossom Bath Oil 65, Soapweed
    Natural Shampoo 69

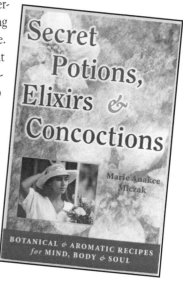

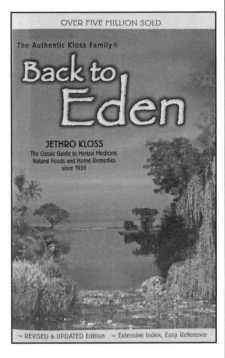

Medicinal Herb Handbook
by Feather Jones, Clinical Herbalist

This book is an extremely handy and useful guide to choosing and utilizing herbs for health and well-being. It focuses on the most commonly called upon herbs and combinations. Its simple reference style gets the information to you quickly and concisely.

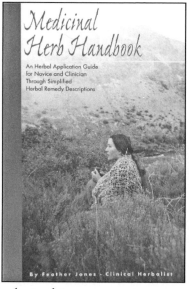

Herbal medicine is finding a niche in the alternative health care field. Earth-centered values and global consciousness are taking the forefront in our resolve to heal the planet of its human-made diseases.

Herbs are a valuable way to maintain and restore health, but they must be respected and used in appropriate ways. They cannot be seen as simply a "standardized active ingredient" (which is essentially what we call a pharmaceutical "drug"), but rather as a wholistic complex of energies and nutrients put together in a way that promotes gentle healing and well-being. By respecting herbs in this way, we gain a new relationship to the plants, the environment, the entire planet that is in itself a healing force in this time of great global environmental dislocation.

Trade Paper   ISBN 978-0-9149-5587-0   40 pp $4.95

Available at bookstores and natural food stores nationwide, or order your copy directly by sending $4.95 plus $2.50 shipping/handling ($.75 s/h for each additional copy ordered at the same time) to:

Lotus Press, P O Box 325, Twin Lakes, WI 53181 USA
toll free order line: 800 824 6396 office phone: 262 889 8561
office fax: 262 889 8591 email: lotuspress@lotuspress.com
web site: www.lotuspress.com

Lotus Press is the publisher of a wide range of books and software in the field of alternative health, including Ayurveda, Chinese medicine, herbology, aromatherapy, Reiki and energetic healing modalities. Request our free book catalog.

Planetary Herbology

by Dr. Michael Tierra

A major work integrating the herbal traditions of the East with those of the West by the bestselling author of "The Way of Herbs". This practical handbook and reference guide is a landmark publication in this field. For unprecedented usefulness in practical applications, the author provides a comprehensive listing of the more than 400 medicinal herbs available in the west, classified according to their chemical constituents, properties and actions, indicated uses and suggested dosages.

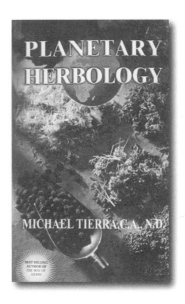

Trade Paper Book   ISBN: 978-0-9415-2427-8   490 pp pb $17.95

Available at bookstores and natural food stores nationwide or order your copy directly by sending $17.95 plus $2.50 shipping/handling ($.75 s/h for each additional copy ordered at the same time) to:

Lotus Press, PO Box 325, Dept. NW, Twin Lakes, WI 53181 USA
toll free order line: 800 824 6396   office phone: 262 889 8561
office fax: 262 889 2461   email: lotuspress@lotuspress.com
web site: www.lotuspress.com

Lotus Press is the publisher of a wide range of books and software in the field of alternative health, including Ayurveda, Chinese medicine, herbology, aromatherapy, Reiki and energetic healing modalities. Request our free book catalog.

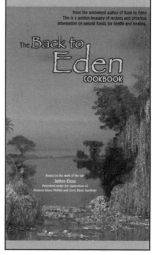

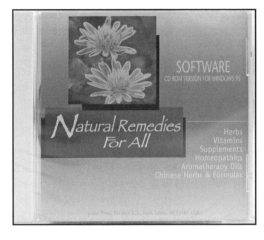

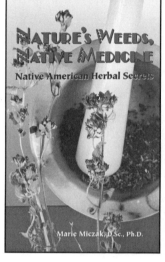